D1252229

Birthing in Good Hands

Birthing in Good Hands

HOLISTIC MASSAGE FOR PREGNANCY, LABOR, AND BABIES

Christine Sutherland, RMT

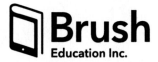
Brush
Education Inc.

Brush Education Inc.
www.brusheducation.ca
contact@brusheducation.ca

Cover and interior design: Carol Dragich.
Cover images: photo of lily from stock.adobe.com; photo of Sarah Murray by Crystal Anielewicz

Proofreading: Shauna Babiuk

Index: Judy Dunlop

Illustrations: Chapter 7 by Brandon Besharah, RMT, illustrator; all others by Chao Yu, Vancouver

All photos by Crystal Anielewicz, Sherri Bennett, Camara Cassin, Peter Schramm, Sarah Yarwood, and Christine Sutherland

Library and Archives Canada Cataloguing in Publication

Sutherland, Christine, 1951-, author
     Birthing in good hands : holistic massage for pregnancy, labor, and babies / Christine Sutherland.

Includes bibliographical references and index.
Issued in print and electronic formats.
ISBN 978-1-55059-744-8 (softcover).--ISBN 978-1-55059-745-5 (PDF).--ISBN 978-1-55059-746-2 (Kindle).--ISBN 978-1-55059-747-9 (EPUB)

     1. Pregnant women--Health and hygiene. 2. Massage therapy.
3. Prenatal care. 4. Postnatal care. 5. Maternal health services. I. Title.

RG525.S875 2018   618.2'4   C2018-901357-5
                                          C2018-901358-3

We acknowledge the support of the Government of Canada
Nous reconnaissons l'appui du gouvernement du Canada | Canadä

Contents

Disclaimer

The publisher, author, contributors, and editors bring substantial expertise to this book and have made their best efforts to ensure it is useful, accurate, safe, and reliable.

Nonetheless, practitioners must always rely on their own experience, knowledge, and judgment when consulting any of the information contained in this book or employing it in patient care. When using any of this information, they should remain conscious of their responsibility for their own safety and the safety of others, and for the best interests of those in their care.

Non-expert users should put safety first at all times. When you are at all uncertain of how to proceed, opt in favour of gentleness and non-intervention. If you have any health or safety concerns, stop and consult a professional.

To the fullest extent of the law, neither the publishers, the author, the contributors, nor the editors assume any liability for injury or damage to persons or property from any use of information or ideas contained in this book.

First Birth

It was 1977. I had driven across the country to be at a home birth after receiving an invitation from a young man named Jim, a former massage student of mine. He called me from northern Ontario to request my attendance at the birth of a woman he had fallen in love with. I didn't hesitate. After giving notice at my job, I drove east, excited to be invited to the birth.

It all seemed right. Right to go east again, right to accept the invitation, right to answer the calling.

I had a place to stay in Toronto at my friend Rose Marie's house on Beverley Street in the heart of the city. That spring, everyone in our house was on alert for a call from the North. Sarilyn, my housemate at Rosie's place, was going to come as well. The woman Jim was in love with, Judy, was Sarilyn's best friend.

The call came early one morning. Judy's water had broken and she was in active labor. Sarilyn and I headed three hours north, my hardy antique Renault climbing the snowy, white hills of Muskoka. We arrived in the backcountry fortified with coffee and sweets from our travels. The cabin looked inviting. Smoke poured out of the chimney as we ran to the door.

We found them in the loft, Jim beside Judy, Judy on her back pushing. I still remember the intense heat. Sarilyn and I were dressed for winter, with turtlenecks, corduroy pants, and long sleeves. We were a colorful contrast to our birthing partners' bare skin and scanty attire in the steamy woodstove warmth.

Jim had a heavy meditative vibe going with Judy that Sarilyn and I dove right into. The air was thick with the essence of relaxation. Sarilyn and I each took up a leg and began massaging Judy's inner thighs. Instinctively, we worked as a team to relax her muscles.

All were full of enthusiasm for this delivery, but none of us had ever seen the birth of a human being.

I had been on call for a dairy near Salmon Arm, in the heart of British Columbia, during calving season about five years earlier. The farmers had called me at my request to attend the birth of a calf. I had

met them on a Saturday morning at the dump, where the farmers congregated to talk farm talk. I was hoping to solicit an opportunity to see life start in a live barnyard birth, and make the course I was taking at the Centre for Human Development more relevant. Our meditations on the birth and death of ideas seemed so abstract when I had no idea what a birth of any kind was about, so I went looking for real life. I went looking for a farmer.

My class caught wind of what I was up to, and when the farmer's call came in, about six of us jumped into a borrowed VW station wagon and tore up the mountain to the dairy farm. We watched the farmer loop ropes around the calf's hooves and work with the mother with each contraction to help pull the calf out. We watched that calf come to life, find its legs, stand, and instinctively look for its mother's milk. We felt intoxicated as we raced back to the rest of our classmates, jubilant with our experience. After that, I attended many barnyard births, but this would be my first human birth.

This time, it was not hooves that were presenting themselves. The rhythmic opening of Judy's cervix revealed a hairy, scrumpled bunch of skin. I thought something was going terribly wrong and I did not know how to break it to Judy that her insides were coming out! I worried about what we were going to do and wished I had taken more first aid courses or read more books or had prepared for labor and delivery with my friends' nursing textbooks.

Not wanting to alarm anyone, I said nothing. Sarilyn and I just kept breathing with Judy, massaging and keeping the energy calm.

Then a head popped out. That hairy skin was actually scalp—a baby's scalp! It blinked and slowly rotated on its own. Now the baby's head was facing Judy's inner thigh and we were waiting for the next contraction. The baby's head looked perfect.

Then I saw a whitish, bluish cord wrapped twice around the baby's neck. Without thinking, I grabbed the cord and slipped my fingers underneath. I loosened its grip and tugged on the part that was still inside Judy. The baby's head was still at the entrance to her birth canal. Sarilyn held Judy's legs as I gently loosened the lasso and the baby slid past his mom's grip.*

He landed in Sarilyn's hands and was immediately transferred into Judy's arms. While she and Jim cuddled their newborn, Sarilyn and I watched for the afterbirth, which delivered without a hitch.

I had seen only cow and goat placentas before. This human placenta was slippery, heavy, and bigger than I had thought it would be: it was huge, like a lung crossed with a liver. It was dark red—nearly black—and purple.

Judy wanted to save it for making stew, so we washed it and put it into the fridge. I then gave Judy a postpartum massage—the postevent sports massage I had learned for hockey players, this time delivered with a feeling of spiritual significance, still in the afterglow of witnessing one of life's major miracles.

Sarilyn and I ran down the hill through the smell of freshly baked bagels coming from one of the neighboring cabins. We took off our clothes and tiptoed through the spring snow to the creek, where we dipped ourselves into the freezing water. Our noisy midwifery celebration joined the surge of the creek, and then we warmed up in the April sun.

It must have looked surreal—our bare skin against a backdrop of white snow, Judy bearing witness as she leaned against the door of the cabin, gracefully transformed, radiant in the afternoon sun.

Today, as I look at the photo of us in the moments after that birth, I can still feel the overwhelming heat of the loft and smell the wood smoke. I still feel the envelope of soft transformation that greeted us as we climbed up the ladder into the embrace of Jim and Judy's transcontinental invitation. I remember the intensity of our arrival on the scene. But most of all, I remember Judy's generosity of spirit and Jim's request for help that combined to give me my start on this wonderful adventure and lifelong career of birthing in good hands.

To all my birthing partners and patients, thank you for bringing me into the intimacy of your births; thank you for teaching me lessons to pass along. Thank you, especially, to my first birthing mom, Judy Pustil; also thank you to my lifelong friend, now international midwifery instructor/midwife, Sarilyn Zimmerman, and our big sister, Rose Marie Harrop, who brought us together. To all of you, I dedicate this book.

---

* Although I didn't know it at the time, midwives have told me it's a myth that the cord wrapped around the baby's neck is necessarily life threatening. Midwives are specifically trained to not worry about the cord and just slip it over the baby's head or slide it down the baby's body. It can be around the neck once, twice, or even three times.

The Power of Touch

Birthing has come full circle.

My mother and grandmother were born at home. In the early fifties, I was born into the modern system of baby arrivals, the first generation of hospital births. Like deaths, births were taken out of the home in the postwar era and put into hospitals and medical settings so that a family no longer experienced the traditional way of arriving and departing.

Now we have choices: to have our babies anywhere and everywhere, at home or in hospital, with medical teams coming to our homes again. Traditional midwives are a "welcome-back" addition to today's deliveries, and now there are new players on the block: doulas. These birthing professionals are worldwide, old style, and New Age. We get the benefits of tradition and choice, plus the wonders of medical technology where it's needed.

After more than forty years helping to deliver babies with midwives, doulas, doctors, husbands, mothers, and grandmothers, I am still in awe of the power of touch to alleviate the aches and pains of one of life's most intense (and magical) experiences.

If we didn't get pregnant with such enthusiasm, if the experience of fertilization wasn't so pleasant, if sex didn't belong to childbirth, we might think twice about procreating! Pregnancy includes a full-body spectrum of maternity conditions, from headaches to sore feet. That list includes shortness of breath as the baby grows bigger; problems of the upper extremities, such as numbness and carpal tunnel syndrome; myriad back problems, including resurrection of old or recent sports injuries of the active mother-to-be; and digestive problems such as constipation and abdominal pressure due to the rearranging of the pelvis. The lower extremities often show contracted iliotibial bands, sciatica, knee problems, spasms in the calf muscles, and flat feet. And then there is the legendary pain of childbirth itself, plus postpartum discomforts, including depression.

If we knew that this experience was coming with hands-on massage remedies for all the uncomfortable parts of the process, if we knew that we were not alone in our discomforts, if we could be guaranteed that we would deliver the goods with ease and less pain, we would be happily pregnant and enthusiastically looking forward to the experience of labor and delivery.

Many pregnancy symptoms are treatable by massage. Massage can be defined as the manipulation of body tissues for therapeutic purposes. Massage has been used since ancient times to treat a variety of ailments, generally with a role in maintaining or restoring a healthy balance to the body.

Touch has the power to heal, calm, and nurture relationships. In 1971, when anthropologist Ashley Montagu published *Touching: The Human Significance of the Skin*, his ideas were considered revolutionary. In *Touching*, Montagu explored the many studies on humans and animals showing the health benefits of good touch. His book gave me the background and research I needed to back up what I already knew about the "mind of the skin."

More recent studies by neuroscientist Edmund Rolls indicates that touch stimulates the part of the brain associated with feelings of pleasure and compassion.[1] Other research shows promise for one day better understanding how massage affects circulation and postworkout recovery.[2] Well-publicized research on children deprived of human touch in Romanian orphanages demonstrates conclusively that touch is essential to human physical, social, and emotional development. Dacher Keltner, a professor of psychology at the University of

California, Berkeley, tells us "the science of touch convincingly suggests that we're wired to—we need to—connect with other people on a basic physical level. To deny that is to deprive ourselves of some of life's greatest joys and deepest comforts."[3]

That massage is helpful in reducing stress, promoting relaxation, and increasing a sense of well-being is well-established. However, exactly *how* and *why* massage has these effects is not well-understood and requires more scientific study. A close review of the scientific literature by Tracy Walton of the Massage Therapy Foundation found that widespread claims that massage reduces cortisol levels (associated with stress), that massage helps the body detoxify, and that massage helps prevent muscle soreness caused by lactic acid have not been definitively proven by solid scientific studies. However, she writes, "That doesn't mean massage doesn't 'work'; it just means it might not work the way we think, or the way we've been taught."[4] Lack of scientific explanations does not negate consistent clinical evidence that massage has positive effects.

One widely accepted study, by Tiffany Field, head of the Touch Research Institute at the Miller School of Medicine in Miami, found that preterm babies given just fifteen minutes of touch therapy a day gain 47 percent more weight than those with traditional medical treatment alone. Field also found that massage therapy reduces prenatal depression and pain in pregnant women, a finding that confirms my own experiences.[5]

My birth stories span many years, from my first birth in the 1970s to my most recent birth last night. They are stories influenced by Ina May Gaskin and Sheila Kitzinger, the Kübler-Rosses of midwifery. I never met Ina May or Sheila in person, but their books, popular in the seventies, were influential in fighting the institutionalization of birth, bringing birthing back into the home and the hands of women.

We were all trying to make a difference in the seventies. I was one of those self-subsistent small-time farmers with sixty chickens, a couple milking goats, some geese, and horses. I thought the world would be a better place if everyone were more environmentally friendly and conscientious, composting, recycling, and looking after their own health. We were New Age "back to the land" pioneers.

My first birth in the backwoods of Ontario was scary. I'll never forget seeing the baby present with the cord around his neck. This first birth was followed by a home birth in which I thought we were going to lose the mom when her blood pressure plummeted. Fortunately, we had a great midwife who kept us calm. I knew I was designed for these kinds of special deliveries when a later patient, whom I was massaging, had to have a C-section and ditched her husband so I could stay with her throughout the surgery. He was relieved; I was thrilled.

In 1978, two years after I met Grace Chan as her instructor at the 3HO School of Massage Therapy in Toronto, we started our own professional massage training program. We were determined to change the world of massage therapy. We wanted to have a school with a two-year program instead of the part-time, one-year programs available at the time. We wanted to double the required massage hours for our students and include an outreach program and student clinic. Our students would have lots of hands-on training by doing at least one hundred massages before graduating.

Five years later, we had grown into another creature with more staff and more patients and more responsibilities. We had graduate clinics, on-site clinics, and busy sports and wheelchair massage groups. I love teaching, so the school was a wonderful arena for me to pass on what I knew from my clinical experience and to train others to teach.

Twelve years passed in a flash, and I now had a baby of my own. Both my husband, Willie, and I owned businesses that were all-consuming. To fit in parenting, we had a system called football baby, in which we passed Crystal back and forth from work site to work site. I would teach Saturday mornings for the public in a class that ended at one o'clock. My husband would spend the mornings with our daughter and pass her to me near the end of my class on his way to work. My classes in basic massage got a special baby-massage half hour at the end. Crystal was a demo baby extraordinaire.

I loved my work, but I knew I would have regrets if I didn't take my daughter west to help with my aging parents in British Columbia. Grace took over the school and clinics and I headed home, where I continued to teach at Selkirk College in Nelson. I also had the opportunity to merge my previous career as an audiovisual specialist with my massage instructor skills. Willie, a computer animation specialist, helped produce many of my early videos, which ranged from baby and pregnancy massage to wheelchair and palliative massage.

Because I had a vocal disorder that didn't allow me to speak easily, I played the films while I circulated in my classroom from table to table. The videos and my interactive teaching techniques allowed me to be vocally impaired and still be a good instructor.

My philosophy of teaching was—and still is—to teach students to be teachers and to pass along what we know to family and friends. Sharing the gift of touch through the maternity massage stories in this book is important to me. If I have a legacy, I want it to be the tried-and-true massage techniques perfected through years of partnership with laboring couples.

My massage practice from the beginning included unique types of pregnancies, such as embryonic transplants, in vitro fertilization, gay pregnancies, communal birthing teams, and everything in between. My work also includes the other end of life, with an intense focus on palliative massage, so my patients arrive and depart at all times of the day and night.

Today more than ever, countries worldwide need hands-on pain management in these same two areas: birthing and dying. There is never going to be an abundance of modern medicine, let alone electricity to run our medical equipment to analyze how the labor and delivery are going and how the baby is doing. Touch has been and always will be a trustworthy foundation for information retrieval in the world of birthing.

Whether I am teaching in Guatemala, Africa, the Cayman Islands, Haiti, or northern Canada,

I team up with local professionals to see what I can contribute and what I can learn. They are my teachers who continue to fuel my passion for passing along the power of touch.

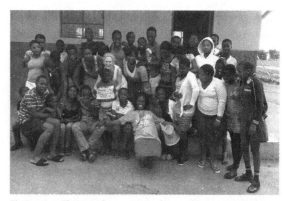

Figure 0.1. This youth group just learned how to give their grandparents head, neck, and shoulder massages—many of the young people had been raised by grandparents after their parents died of AIDS. I was helped by the staff at the Stephen Lewis Foundation Hospice in Durban, South Africa.

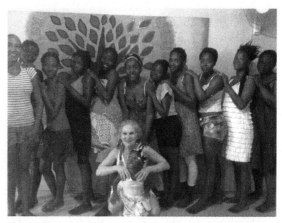

Figure 0.2. In 2014, the midwifery students at the Olive Tree Birthing Center in Haiti included their pregnant patients in the head, neck, and shoulder massage lessons, with me demonstrating on my four-year-old volunteer.

In 2007 in Guatemala, most of the midwives I taught were elderly. Their experienced hands were worn and wizened; their touch was golden. They showed me the techniques for labor and delivery that had been used for hundreds of years birthing babies in their villages. These seniors were maternity grandmothers, with ancient birthing methods combined with superstitions and myths.

In 2017, when I taught at a midwifery school in Guatemala City, I was the oldest in the class. One other person was over fifty and the rest of the students were between twenty and twenty-five. What fascinated me was their appetite for learning, despite their already rich inheritance of traditional midwifery. Until now, they had used traditional pressure by binding the back with long cummerbunds that would help the woman in her squatting posture for delivery. My suggestion to use counterpressure on the low back to help the pain of contractions was immediately taken up by the midwives, even though they had no massage in their birthing protocols. I was impressed by how open they were to change. Through all my travels, it seems that only in North America do we undervalue what our hands know how to do.

Slowly, researchers are catching up to what wise hands have known for decades. In 1999, twenty-six pregnant women were assigned to either a massage-therapy or a relaxation-therapy group for five weeks. The therapies consisted of twenty-minute sessions twice a week. Both groups reported feeling less anxious after the first session and having less leg pain after the first and last sessions. Only the massage-therapy group, however, reported reduced anxiety, improved mood, better sleep, and less back pain by the last day of the study. In addition, stress-hormone levels decreased for the massage-therapy group, and the women had fewer complications during labor. Their infants also had fewer postnatal complications.[6]

In another study from 2014, thirty women with low back pain received ten sessions of either massage therapy or physical therapy. Although both groups experienced decreased pain and greater range of motion, the effects were greater for the massage-therapy group.[7]

Neuroscientist David Linden, from Johns Hopkins University, is on the forefront of medical research into pain management through touch. He says that "Right now, we have good drugs to blunt pain, but with terrible side effects. But what if we could just *block* pain, without the euphoria of things like morphine or the bowel disruption of so

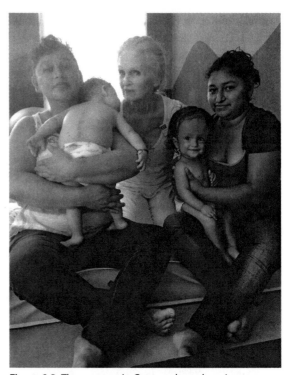

Figure 0.3. These moms in Guatemala are learning to massage their babies with special needs. One baby is listless and the other is hydrocephalic (enlarged head) with little muscles holding up a heavy head. The listless baby was stimulated from the massages right away.

many medicines?"[8] Researchers are excited about possibilities for pain management to be found in new research looking at the genes common to our touch and pain receptors.

As a medical professional, I want to help shift the world of maternity and palliative pain management. The power of touch, our ancient medicine, put in the hands of the suffering public, will make the uncomfortable transitions of life more comfortable.

Pregnancy deserves daily massage as a reprieve from the symptoms of the growing baby. Pregnant women can have an army of helpers (husbands, siblings, mothers, mothers-in-law, girlfriends, and boyfriends) for any symptoms of pregnancy that take away from the pleasure of carrying a new life.

We can teach children to massage their siblings in utero. We can learn to massage our friends during labor and delivery and be part of the delivery team in hospitals or homes. I have seen how massage done by the average nonprofessional makes an enormous difference in arrivals of all kinds, even with special deliveries through C-section or prolonged back labor.

Massage can also help keep partners in tune with one another. This book includes easy head, neck, and shoulder massages that pregnant women can give to their partners prenatal and postnatal. Keeping in touch with each other during pregnancy, labor, delivery, and postpartum is a lifeline for both parents. Massages, even if brief, remind the couple of their original enthusiasm for touching each other. In the most consuming of "after-birth" circumstances, such as postpartum depression or surgery, that special touch is the calming, reassuring, and loving gesture that will bring good energy to an otherwise challenging situation.

Readers wanting to learn baby massage are in a contemporary classroom of massage enthusiasts that may include siblings, grandparents, and dads (or other birth partners). Zoomer baby massage is becoming popular with lots of grandparents on the frontlines. I now have baby massage classes just for dads and grandparents.

Men, in particular, are changing the world of maternity massage. They are eager to learn pregnancy massage, labor and delivery massage, and baby massage. They are changing gender tactile boundaries and my experience as a teacher.

These dads can be a challenge to teach as they sometimes arrive knowing everything already, each one in his wonderful unique maleness. They have read up on massage for everything. They know how to do pregnancy massage Thai style, baby massage New-Age style, and they have watched more videos on labor and delivery than I would have thought possible. Some have already watched all my YouTube videos. But these are the right kind of know-it-alls.

Keeping the men involved with skin-on-skin contact for both the mother and the new baby is important for the recipients of his touch as well as, as the research shows, for the husband himself, reducing his anxiety and improving domestic bliss.

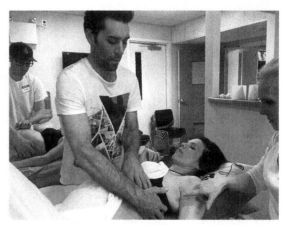

Figure 0.4. Serious dads, serious rib raking at the Apple Tree Maternity Clinic in Nelson, British Columbia.

When I ask fathers how they think massage will help their marriages, they are quick to respond with predictable answers. But what struck me about working with these partners is their genuine enthusiasm for having a worthwhile job to do during the pregnancy.

These new dads then teach their kids what to do with second babies. They also teach one another. My most wonderful memory of teaching baby massage was listening to one dad tell the other, "Christine taught us to do the side-lying position this way, but I found over the last few days it's easiest to do it my way." The fact that he'd massaged his baby so much that he'd developed his own way of doing things was so rewarding. After more than forty years of teaching baby massage, that was my biggest payoff.

I live in the small town of Nelson, in the heart of British Columbia, where men push the majority of the baby carriages on our streets. These men meet in coffee shops and run along the waterfront in the early morning with their babies. My baby-massage classes have more dads than ever before, and through the quick exchange of information today, men are becoming expert Internet dads long before their babies arrive. This current generation is the new frontier of baby massagers. These young parents are keen to be shown hands-on techniques for birthing perfect babies.

Kids with special needs have always been a favorite part of my massage practice. Babies with Down's syndrome, babies that are premature or delayed, palliative pediatrics, and babies with cystic fibrosis or cerebral palsy are all ideal candidates for hands-on massage therapy. I have learned some of my best massage techniques from the parents of special-needs kids. They are the people truly invested in daily therapy. We are racing to catch up with their skills and rewrite our textbooks.

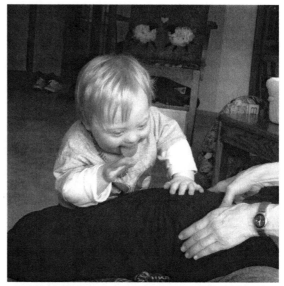

Figure 0.5. We usually focus on how to massage our special-needs kids the right way, but here a toddler learns to massage his postpartum mom.

TWO MOTHERS, TWO DAUGHTERS

The night I went into labor, people began to gather. Our midwife, Margaret, arrived from out of town. Our doctor arrived and they both examined me and discussed their findings. It seems that the baby was not large but was bumped up against my pelvis the wrong way. They agreed that things would probably right themselves naturally.

Margaret promised to call the doctor with updates. My husband, Willie, was a natural at responding to my pain with his hands-on skills. However, he found that he was using his feet more than his hands. Willie's foot on my sacrum eased the pressure and discomfort in my low back dramatically.

The next morning, my birthing team arrived. First Gail, later Jane, and then Trish. I was in good hands.

It was October 1st and warm and sunny. I was able to labor in the garden on my back with my team of women, but things were not progressing. When I was examined by my midwife and she talked about my coccyx getting in the way, I remembered that I broke my tailbone in a horse accident. The baby was not turning in the way it was supposed to, to line up for delivery, so I was on my side with everyone working to get the baby to realign. The massages were relieving and rejuvenating.

By that night, we were staggering around the neighborhood in the dark. I would have a contraction and Willie would hold on to me in the middle of the kids' playground next to the grocery store. I really wanted to kneel on the ground, but he kept me vertical. The idea was that this vertical stroll could get the baby's head lower and stretch my cervix. I seemed to be stuck at three inches (8 cm) forever.

The fact that our baby was posterior was now obvious as my back pain never let up between contractions. The baby's spine was lying against my spine instead of sticking out to the front of me. The pressure seemed unbearable. I could tolerate the steady discomfort as long as someone had hands on me. I had been in active labor now for over twenty hours. I was bordering on delirium by midnight. All night long, I labored and the decision was reached that if all our big plans to turn this baby around did not work, then we were heading to the hospital.

I did all the hula dancing and side-lying I could do. I had learned about all the natural ways that babies like to come down the chute, but this baby was stuck. It figures! In my massage practice, I had attended every kind of delivery that I had ever imagined. Now I was experiencing my own special delivery.

Somewhere around two in the morning, I punched Willie in the shoulder (deltoid to be exact) when he asked me to breathe deeply. I was kneeling on my hands and knees beside him and I watched myself haul back and punch him. I didn't know why I did that. It was nothing to do with him, just to do with the pain.

"Christine, you just punched me."

"I know, I'm so sorry. I didn't mean to punch you."

Willie picked up the phone when I started to moan that I wanted my mother. I was in the bathtub at the time. My mom talked me down.

"You're doing a great job. Willie is right there for you. Don't worry. The baby will come soon. No matter what, the baby will come! Just let everyone help you through."

Of course I had hoped for a home birth. But after thirty-six hours in labor and twenty-four hours of back labor, I opted for the hospital, where my husband continued to massage me through an epidural and a high forceps delivery. I knew that this was a special delivery when my business partner, Grace, appeared like an apparition as I lay on my side, almost passed out from the epidural relaxation, her face close to mine whispering that my inlaws were in the lobby of the birthing center in hysterics and that she would try to keep them calm. There was an explosion when the doors of the operating room burst open and Willie's dad ran in with the security guard on his heels. He circled the room, spotted me, and darted in for a kiss and pat to his grandchild before the officer picked him up and hauled him out of the green tiled room.

Crystal was born a tiny five pounds, five ounces. She was calm, sleeping, and comfortable. She was delivered not only by me but by an invisible stork. This was not the advertising stork with the handkerchief in its beak, flying through the air, making graceful deliveries. This stork landed on Crystal's head! She had baby bruises just above her eyes and on the back of her head. They called them stork marks. That friendly touch of flight into this life.

I had never experienced such powerful sensations in all of my other painful experiences like breaking bones, falling off ladders, being burned and beaten. This was unlike anything else. It was as though I had experienced some horrific trauma of delightful proportion—like dying, but I had recovered and come back to life. Restored and reborn.

I had hands-on help all the way, with footprints on my back from Willie's pressure. I had stitches to prove my worth and had come back from the war of the womb to tell the tale. My discomfort was bearable through the help I received during that challenging birth. I could have never endured the pain had I not been massaged by the team of friends that attended me at home, in the garden, walking the street throughout the nights, and finally in the hospital!

Now my baby girl has a baby of her own. Paige has arrived, bigger than her mother, but shorter in labor and delivery. The circle of life completed itself. Watching Crystal and her partner Joel birth Paige brought Crystal's birth around the corner of time.

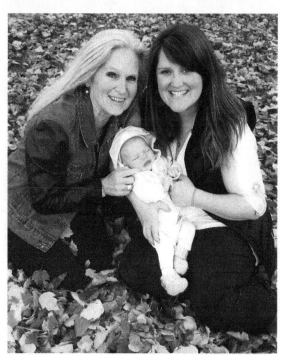

Figure 0.6. Three generations, 2015: Christine, Crystal, and Paige.

I am no longer just a mother. I am a grandmother. Crystal and I are now forever two mothers sharing two deliveries birthing two daughters.

The power of touch can change the world, simply by raising our children with massage as a way of life. These are the kids and the generation that can change the world. These kids will take it to the streets with their hugs in school, their hands on their grandparents, and their general comfort with touching. We can take this message of hands-on healing to the streets, with events like Massage Mondays and flash-mob massages at local hospitals, where people can use their massage skills to bring comfort to the most demanding work environments. The kids we are raising need massage and loving touch from their first breath to their first scary moment.

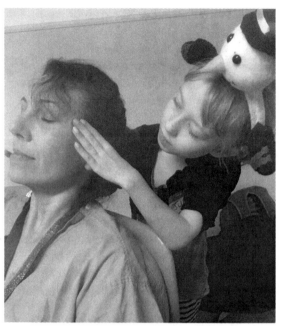

Figure 0.8. Jupiter's experience with massage began in utero, after her family learned massage for pregnancy, labor, and delivery. She has volunteered since she was four years old at the BC Seniors Games massaging dragon boat teams. Now seven, she is seen here in the flash-mob massage for hospital staff in Nelson, British Columbia.

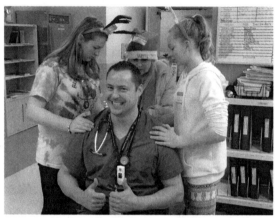

Figure 0.7. Boxing Day flash-mob massage for the medical staff at the Fort St. John Hospital, 2017. The hospital staff receive hands-on thank yous from the students from the local middle school performing community volunteer work.

Whether baby massage is used in orphanages, institutions, daycare centers, or family homes, it is a traditional, ancient medical art again becoming contemporary. The return to our original medical practices of hands-on therapy using the power of touch to soothe, stimulate, repair, nurture, and cultivate closeness is even more needed today. Families are where social change takes place. In doing daily massages, those shoulder rubs around the kitchen table, we give the most love in the best way.

This book is for medical professionals, such as nurses, physiotherapists, and massage therapists. It's equally for people with no medical training but who are eager to learn to touch with skill and compassion. I believe everyone deserves high-quality pregnancy, labor and delivery, and postpartum care through the gift of touch, whether they receive it through professionals and institutions or through friends and family. Through the stories, instructions, photos, and illustrations in this book, join me in birthing the world into better hands.

1

Pregnancy Massage Basics

This book covers massage for every stage of bringing a new baby into the world, from the massages leading to pregnancy to the baby massages so important to parental bonding and baby thriving.

This chapter begins with the basic strokes and equipment you will need. Chapter 2 helps you learn massage techniques for each trimester of pregnancy, and chapter 3 suggests specific massage treatments of some of the most common conditions in pregnancy. Chapter 4 deals with labor and delivery, and chapter 5 gives massage for the physical and emotional needs of the postpartum phase. Chapter 6 explains how to massage for the challenges of breastfeeding, and chapter 7 gets you set up for the most fun of all: massaging your new baby!

Role of Massage in Pregnancy

In a typical healthy pregnancy, there is much to treat with massage therapy, from the discomfort of prenatal headaches to flat feet. Low back pain, digestive troubles, and respiratory tension are the most common complaints in the body of a pregnant woman. Added body weight and extra fluid in the extremities give rise to carpal tunnel syndrome and numbness in the fingers. The lower extremities sport the conditions of sciatica, contracted iliotibial bands, knee problems, spasms in the calves, swollen ankles, and foot cramping.

Massage is the best way to get feedback from your body even before you are pregnant. I always encourage couples to look at the year of getting pregnant as preparing for a major sports event. Signing up for the race is a commitment to be as strong as possible for the event. Anyone can train for success if they have enough time and a good team to help keep them on track.

The Maternity Team

The most common maternity team is made up of the core players that make the event happen in the first place: the couple working to get pregnant. But there are others to invite into this inner sanctum at the beginning of the marathon. Usually, the people we inform first become important players on our maternity team. When I found out I was pregnant, I told my husband first, and then our parents and best friends. I knew my team would be these people, those who would be there for me, hands on at every stage.

Over the years, I have worked with an incredible variety of birthing teams. One patient, a single mother having her fourth child, had a wonderful family and mother who all showed up to the labor room. When I arrived, it looked like a family reunion with seven adults and three children talking and laughing in excitement. I quickly got the mob under control and focused by giving them each a hands-on job to do. To this day, that is still my biggest team.

I've had a transgender couple, gay couples, single moms, adopting parents, giving-up-for-adoption moms, and surrogate moms; they all had their own special teams of people. I once had a best man massaging his friend's wife in the final month of her pregnancy. I've also had many lesbian couples, who sometimes involve their other single lesbian friends; for many, this is the only birth they may ever experience. When my patients Selena and Julie had Dénali, there were so many female couples at that baby's celebration, it seemed like a women's festival.

Although the people on your team might not be instinctively good at doing massage, they share your joy and enthusiasm for the new baby. I am always surprised at the efforts families make to become comfortable massaging the pregnant woman. With the right feedback about their touch, even the most ungifted tactile types can be taught to listen and feel with a touch that is not only therapeutic but also relaxing. Never underestimate the power of family for helping throughout the pregnancy and then through the miracle of labor and delivery.

My mom was very good with her hands. My father was also a hands-on person. Together they gave me the gift of touch. Even though she couldn't be with me when I gave birth to my daughter, my mom came to mind when I was in the throes of despair in my labor. I talked with her on the phone from the bathtub; I cried for her as I was wheeled down the hospital corridor; from across the country, she was with me in my moments of pain. She was still on my team, even from a distance.

Just last year, I taught my daughter's fiancé, Joel, to do the massages for her second trimester in a tandem massage tutorial. He has a natural touch. I felt inspired and confident that I was leaving her in good hands when I saw how quickly he picked up her feedback and adapted his strokes to suit her.

So many pregnant women could benefit from daily massages but don't have people with available hands to work on them. Sometimes pregnant partners are working away from home or simply are not the helpful hands-on type. I would like to see a buddy system for pregnancy involving volunteers, especially in the senior age group, who would be available to regularly massage moms-to-be. The latest reports from Statistics Canada show there are, for the first time, more seniors than youth in the country. Let's put those experienced hands to work as partners in maternity massage.

Whatever the maternity massage team looks like, this book will help them be more comfortable being hands on during the pregnancy. Everyone is capable of learning basic massage skills.

Conceiving in Good Hands

The most important massage in the pregnancy story is the conception massage that gets everything off to a good start. Those marathon massages are ways to make the getting-pregnant session extra special. There is never too much massage for getting babies started!

The massage techniques used for pregnancy are also good for encouraging conception. I encourage couples wanting to get pregnant to make some changes to their normal bedtime massaging by checking in with each other about favorite massage strokes. Usually couples, young or old, think they know how to work with their partner because they are so used to each other. I ask them to pretend they are not that familiar, that they are fresh and new to the touch. This freshness is usually, for most, a marriage-enriching idea.

In my work with pregnant couples over the decades, I have found that most people learn massage because they want to be great parents. With that focus, they are eager to learn how to get the baby here in the best way possible. The tactile tone set in pregnancy carries over to the voice of the new family. The act of helping to soothe the symptoms of pregnancy casts a spell over the life of the couple forever, and they carry forward that same loving touch to the next generation they are creating. I am certain that the world changes from massage done during gestation.

How can we get better at pleasing each other, at relaxing each other, and attending to each other's everyday aches and pains? This is the phase of maternity massage that is as creative as the two people making love. Opportunities for bonding, loving, and procreating are right at the tips of our fingers.

The power of touch is also useful in the disappointments that accompany many couples through months and years without fertilization. I don't use the word *unsuccessful* with the sometimes painfully long process of trying to get pregnant. I have worked with many couples who are infertile and never experience childbirth. I am inspired by their level of commitment to massaging each other and, in effect, softening the harshness of those continual disappointments. Their power of touch for each other helps them thrive as a couple and stay emotionally healthy throughout a difficult time.

IN VITRO PREGNANCIES

Although all pregnancies can be stressful in their own way, many women experience a special kind of stress with trouble conceiving and carrying a baby to term. Thankfully modern medicine has given us new options that have helped many couples have the children they desire. I've been fortunate to work with several women who have conceived through in vitro fertilization.

I treated Nancy, a favorite patient of mine, through five special pregnancies. By her fifth in vitro pregnancy, she had one son, Michael, and had three pregnancies that ended in loss. With this history, she was understandably worried about her new pregnancy. She wrote to me, "My strongest memories are of the times I was concerned about the status of the pregnancy and what would result (especially after several difficulties). You always calmed me either with your hands or your heart (or both), providing confidence and reassurance that the world was okay and the child would be fine. You were right. Today, Joseph and Michael are wonderful adults doing very well."

Every time I massaged Nancy, I felt like I was helping with the miracle of her high-tech pregnancy by simply keeping her steady. She is a resilient person, even through heartbreak. I admire her persistence, her bond with her husband, and most of all, her determination to be a mom.

The Maternity Training Program

We should have a workout program for conception. It would look like a training program for any other athlete. People would sign up for the event, grab a bag of massage gear, and head out to the training field. In this case, training would include massage, special baths, and lots of yoga and cardio exercise, especially swimming. I highly recommend swimming before and during pregnancy as a way to keep fit and be gentle on joints like the knees.

A good program to strengthen the abdominal muscles would also be key. Some pregnant women work to develop their abdominal muscles during pregnancy even though they didn't before they became pregnant. There is such a rush to achieve a flat tummy postpartum that many women start early. Working on abdominal strength is great for those with low back pain. Abdominal exercises help strengthen and stabilize the low back and reduce the risk of developing back pain.

Women would get a coach or training partner and would set some goals and a timetable to achieve the strengthening needed in time for the big event. The training partner could be a pregnant friend or someone who just wants to be on the birthing team. Best yet, the woman's conception partner would go running, go swimming, do yoga, and attend weekly pregnancy-massage classes, just to be in shape for new parenthood.

Massage Gear

You don't need much in the way of special equipment for massage. You probably already have most of what you need.

Lubricant

Almost any viscous substance will do as a lubricant, as long as it is healthy: choose one that is edible and nourishing to the skin. Almond oil and cold pressed virgin olive oil are excellent, although they can stain your linens. Nonstaining oils, such as walnut and coconut, are also excellent. I've used coconut oil throughout my massage career. I used to find it only in health food stores, but today it's readily available at nearly every grocery store. If the mom likes fragrances and doesn't have any

A word of caution that aromatherapy is its own form of medicine, and it is always good to research these powerful additives before liberally adding them to your baths or massage oils. I find that the facial creams my daughter suggests for her aging mother register in my taste buds after only a few minutes on my face. Be careful to check your sources and the effects of the specific oils before trying them out.

allergies or sensitivities, you might want to try aromatherapy oils and lotions.

Table

Massage tables are easily available from retail stores and online, but they are not a prerequisite to doing a great home massage. Your bed is fine. The bed is the place most pregnancies start and the place where many babies are born. I have the stature of a twelve-year-old, so I find it easy to move around on the top of a bed to do a massage. However, you might find it easier to stand beside the bed. Some beds today are so high that only a pole-vaulter can access them easily. But these high beds do make it easier for tall people who find it hard to squat or kneel on the bed while massaging.

If the bed seems too awkward, your dining room or kitchen table might be perfect, or you can massage on the living room rug. On a hard surface, lay down something soft, such as a couple yoga mats, to create a comfortable surface for the mom to lie on for about an hour.

Ice massage

I sometimes advocate using ice to treat uncomfortable maternity conditions and old, yet still uncomfortable, injuries. I use the edge of an ice cube to massage, or I make ice popsicles. Using a popsicle tray with pointed shapes to the cones, embed a facecloth at the thickest end of the stem and leave the rest hanging loose. Use the pointed end of the

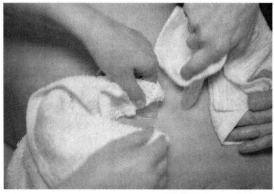

Figure 1.1. Ice popsicles can be useful tools in your pre- and postpregnancy massage repertoire. If you don't want to make a popsicle, hold an ice cube using a facecloth.

popsicle to massage and the loose end of the facecloth to mop up the melting ice as you go. Although you may not need ice popsicles until much later in the pregnancy, I have included the description here since many couples have told me they wish they'd known how to use them earlier.

EPSOM SALT BATHS

I recommend an Epsom salt bath after massage or each night before bed. Salt baths are great for general relaxation, as well as for hemorrhoidal or postnatal discomfort. Epsom salts are readily available at pharmacies, garden centers, farming supply stores, and shopping outlets. I encourage my pregnant patients to buy fifty-pound bags and get someone else to load them into the car and then into their home.

Use about two medium yogurt containers (approximately four cups) of salt for each bath. Add the salt to a few inches of tepid water, and then gradually heat the bath up by adding warmer water. Submerge up to the top of your chest. Place a cold towel around your neck to equalize the temperature in your head and keep you comfortable.

Soak for twenty minutes to one hour.* Don't add any other bathing solutions, oils, or soap since these will alter the chemistry of the water. Never use peppermint oil or any other pure carminative oils since they may irritate or burn mucus membranes.

Drink lots of water. To replenish the fluids you lose as you sweat, keep a large glass of cold water handy on the side of the tub to sip during the bath.

To finish, turn on the shower to rinse off the salts. Slowly turn the water to cooler and cooler. Finish by standing in front of the faucet and letting cool water run down the back of your legs for your puffy feet. Be sure to get out of the bath slowly and carefully. Sit on the edge of the tub to stabilize yourself before getting out.

*Note: Take care not to get overheated. Research indicates that extended overheating of a mother's body can be harmful for the fetus. Consult your doctor for any restrictions or cautions about taking warm or hot baths during your pregnancy.

Other preparation

You will want lots of towels and pillows to support the mom in different massage postures. Keep a stack of towels and five or six pillows at the ready. There are now fancy body pillows that can help support the mom comfortably, but this isn't necessary, as you can easily get enough pillow support with regular pillows.

You will also want a couple hot water bottles, heating pads, or microwavable bean bags. I like to warm the mom's feet and neck while working on other parts of her body. If the mom has an especially tight area, you might want to warm up the area before massage.

The mom can wear a bikini if you want to massage outdoors, or she might wear nothing if you're massaging in private. Use a sheet as a cover to keep her warm or to keep the sun off.

Play music in the pregnancy massages that you can use later in early labor. Getting the brain to associate intense relaxation with certain music is a handy tool for the intensity of labor. For some people, this music is classical or New Age, while others want country ballads or rock and roll. Try the combined favorites of both partners.

Massage to Prevent Stretch Marks

My breasts were my first indication of confirmed pregnancy. It seemed like they popped out the moment I conceived! By my third trimester, they were three times their normal size. By the time I was in my seventh month, I was leaking at the slightest provocation.

Such growth in the breasts and abdomen is often faster than the skin can keep up to. The swelling is uncomfortable, the skin taut. The skin stretches and sometimes tears along the lines of tension, resulting in stretch marks.

Some people are more prone to stretch marks than others. Some of my pregnant patients have no sign of stretch marks in any of their pregnancies, while other moms get stretch marks in the first trimester. Taking steps to prevent stretch marks is especially important for women who have already

seen their bodies produce stretch marks from growth spurts during puberty.

Self-massage is an easy way to help the skin's elasticity and prevent stretch marks. I recommend massage using coconut oil and Vitamin E. You can get the vitamin oil by poking a Vitamin E capsule with a pin and squirting it onto your body. Spread the oil all around the edges of the breasts and lower abdomen and anywhere else it is needed at potential growth and tear sites. Do lots of massage to ease the tension and use lots of oil as your lubricant.

The best stretch mark story advocating therapeutic oils was told to me by Joni, an eighty-six-year-old mother of six. She told me that during the final month of her fourth pregnancy, a Russian neighbor in Grahamdale, Manitoba, brought her goose grease made from rendering the fat from Canada geese (illegal now, but not sixty years ago). The neighbor showed Joni how to massage the odorless and easily absorbed grease into her skin twice a day.

Joni continued this self-massage throughout her last month of pregnancy with great results. The stretch marks from her other three pregnancies were already present, but the goose grease made sure there were no additional stretch marks with her next three babies. Her biggest baby was nearly eleven pounds, and the goose grease saved Joni's stomach from additional stretching and tearing. Today, she still talks about the value of goose grease for making her tummy and breasts more elastic. This elasticity is what we are trying to achieve with our massages all the way through the pregnancy and throughout the breastfeeding months that follow.

Massage Length

Most professional massages run about an hour in length, which is ideal for a full-body massage if you can manage it. However, home massages do not need to be as long. It's better that you do many short, daily massages rather than infrequent hour-long massages. I say the more massages the better, even if each is only a half hour long. On the other hand, a prepregnancy conception massage might be two (or more) hours long!

Principles of Massage

Over my years of teaching and practice, I don't have many massage rules that haven't been modified, changed, or simply ignored when they did not turn out to be true in real life. However, there are a few basic principles I always follow.

1. Uncork the bottle.

The key massage principle here is working from the area closest to the trunk of the body to the farthest away from the trunk. I call it uncorking the bottle. Think of it like this: if you want to get the contents out of a bottle, you need to uncork it first. So always work the part of the extremity (arm or leg) that is hooked up with the trunk of the body first before moving down the length of the extremity. So massage the shoulder first and then the upper arm and then the lower arm. It's the same with the legs: massage the hips first, then the thigh, and then the calf.

Loosen up the area at the top of the arm or leg first. This makes sense for having what is below that area be able to drain up and out of the extremity more easily. The principle of working shoulder to fingers and hips to toes is sound in terms of circulatory theory.

---

2. Apply pressure toward the heart.

One principle of massage I always use is based on the way blood travels around the body. The heart is the pump of the circulatory system. It gives the blood a big push from the center of the body out to our arms and legs, right to the tips of our fingers and toes. These extremities must then work against gravity to return blood to the heart, so our veins are designed with little one-way valves like gates to keep blood moving in the right direction.

Although you start at the trunk and move out to the extremity, the *pressure* of each stroke must always go toward the heart. Your massage pressure

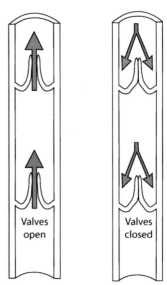

Figure 1.2. Veins have one-way valves that open as the heart beats, permitting blood to flow through, and then close between heartbeats, stopping the blood from moving backward. These valves keep blood moving toward the heart.

always works with the natural blood flow of the body, not against it. Don't push downward with any stroke, whether it be your starting general strokes or the nitty-gritty of therapeutic pressure—each stroke of pressure should go in an upward direction, always toward the heart.

3. Move from general strokes to local strokes and then back to general strokes.

Massage strokes include some superficial, general, large strokes and other smaller, focused, and intense strokes. The superficial strokes tend to smooth out and soothe, while the local strokes really get in and work out tight spots, decreasing contractures and increasing mobility. A massage routine should always start with general strokes, move to specific strokes, and then move back out to general strokes.

Beginning with the general strokes allows the body to adjust and prepare for the therapeutic application of deep tissue release. You want to get the body used to your touch and you want to command the attention of the nervous system to the part being massaged before you work into it.

If I start work on a sore spot too fast, the body will repel me—no thanks!—and then I can get locked out.

So you want to make contact and take the superficial tension off before you work on the underlying tightness. This approach ensures you can get into the problem with a welcoming opening.

After giving a sore or tight spot focused attention, I always end with general strokes that erase the memory of the deeper, stronger strokes. I learned this in the barnyard where I worked with all sorts of injured animals. I always left each animal I worked on with a stroke memory that was positive, not necessarily therapeutic. If the animal remembered me as the one making it uncomfortable, even if there was later therapeutic gain, then it was going to be a lot harder to repeat the treatment. The animal would take one look at me coming into the barn and head for the other side of the stall. So I learned early to "trick" the tissues and leave a lasting impression of positive contact. Leave the area of treatment with the same introductory strokes you started with. As I did with injured horses, you want to leave the tissues happy to see you again.

4. Work both sides.

Another principle is to balance your massage on both sides of the body. People tend to have a favored side to rest on and may not want to lie on the other side very long. Still to this day, I find it hard to ask a comfortable pregnant patient to turn to her uncomfortable side. But even if you can only massage the disfavored side for a brief time, massaging both sides helps bring the person into balance.

Basic Anatomy

Professional massage therapists have extensive knowledge of anatomy, which is critical for solid therapeutic massage. However, you can apply effective massages at home with a basic knowledge of human anatomy. The illustration that follows on page 16 provides some of the basic anatomic knowledge and vocabulary you will find helpful as you work through the massages in this book.

HELPFUL TERMS

Posterior: back	Transverse: across
Anterior: front	Prone: face down
Proximal: close	Supine: face up
Distal: far	Lateral: side

Basic Massage Strokes

Effleurage

Effleurage is a French term that means to cover or cloak. Fittingly, this stroke is most often used to cover or spread the body with oil. It is a warm-up stroke with a gentle, double-loop shape. An introductory stroke, it's the one I use most often to get my hands accustomed to my patient and the patient accustomed to my touch. Effleurage also has its own standalone merits of promoting better circulation. The stroke encourages the superficial circulation to move more effectively, helping to reduce swollen legs or stress and helping to induce relaxation.

To begin a back massage, put some oil or lotion on your hands. It is important to get the right amount of oil, which may take some practice. You want enough oil to provide ease of movement, but not enough to make the person's back slippery. You want your hands to have good contact and not just skate over the surface. Start with just a few drops (not a dollop) and then add more as needed. You don't need to put on the total amount of oil you will use throughout the massage at the beginning. You can add lotion as the massage progresses. If you get too much, towel some off.

Place one hand on each side of the spine, applying firm, even pressure. Use the whole palmar surface of your hands, including fingers: don't be dainty! Keep your fingers together but flat: effleurage is a flat-handed stroke.

Move your hands together from the shoulders down to the low back. At the base of the spine, loop your hands out to the outer back/sides and continue the pressure as you return along the length of the torso to the shoulders. Be firm, especially on the return stroke up the sides. At the shoulders, begin the stroke again. Introductory effleurage

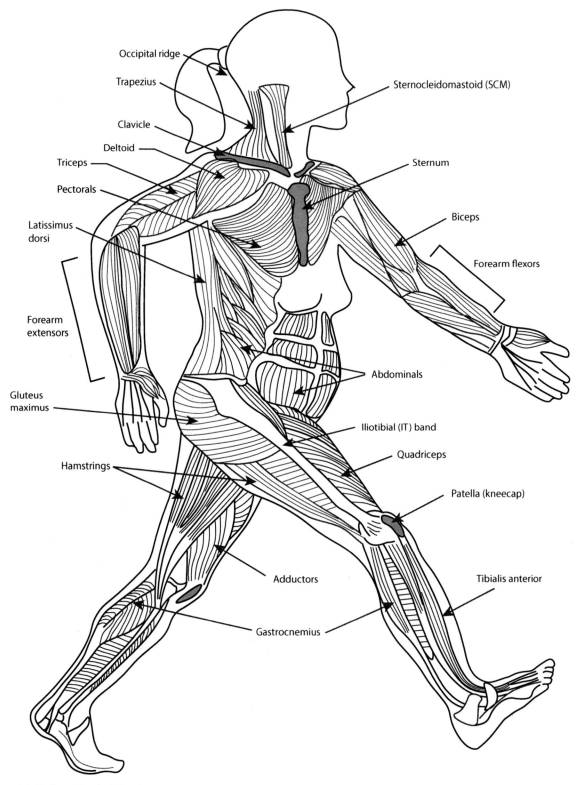

Figure 1.3. Basic anatomical structures.

strokes are done at least three times. The first time spreads the oil, the second time allows you to get comfortable with the stroke, and the third time establishes pressure and gets the circulation moving.

Be sure to check the pressure of your touch with the person you're massaging. Ask if you should apply more or less pressure. Most people are too light in their effleurage strokes.

Remember: when effleuraging the arms or legs, always push up, toward the heart, and never down. You must apply pressure only on the way up and no pressure on the way down, just a light touch. On the back it doesn't matter—you can apply pressure in both directions. The heart is near the middle of the body and the circulatory system is more deeply buried, so the venous return is not directly affected by your direction of pressure.

As this is the beginning of the massage routine, this stroke gives you lots of information about the part of the body you are going to get to know and to accustom the mom to your touch. As your hands warm up, you may be able to feel areas of tension or sensitivity on her body.

I love this stroke. Effleurage is what to do in between other strokes. When you don't know what else to do, effleurage! During pregnancy, this stroke is especially appreciated on the legs because of prenatal swelling and fluid retention. It offers a quick, yet powerful, way to improve circulation and reduce swelling.

I will sometimes talk about a *mini-effleurage*. This is a stroke that covers half or less of the surface covered in a full effleurage. For example, you do a mini-effleurage to start a foot massage, but a full effleurage on the whole leg. You might also use it to start the abdominal massage by effleuraging only the abdominal area, leaving out the breasts, or on the shoulders and neck to begin a head, neck, and shoulder massage.

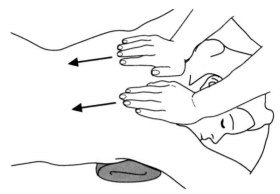

a. Place palms on shoulders.

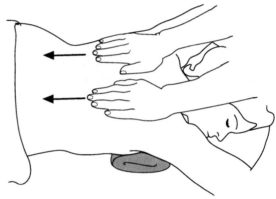

b. Proceed down the erector spinae muscles beside the spine.

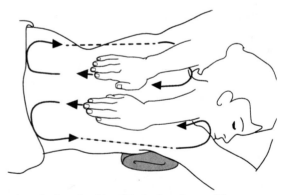

c. Loop back up the sides of the body and around the shoulders to the starting position at the top of the trapezius muscles.

Figure 1.4. Effleurage (at least 3x). On the back, you can use firm pressure both ways.

Wringing

The next two major types of strokes—wringing and kneading—are collectively known as petrissage. If effleurage helps surface tension dissipate, petrissage strokes are more specific and deep reaching in their therapeutic effect. I usually do wringing after effleurage, and then move on to the really focused kneading strokes.

Wringing moves the muscles around more vigorously. It moves the skin away from the underlying muscles to encourage the layers of the tissues to not adhere so tightly to each other. Wringing is another general stroke that helps establish or restore tolerance for more focused, uncomfortable strokes of the thumbs and fingertips. Wringing lengthens muscles by working transversely (across) the tissue. It is an exception to my general practice of massaging in the same direction the muscle fibers run.

On the back, for example, work at right angles to the spine and move your hands in opposition: one hand pushes the skin and underlying flesh away from you around the curve of the ribs, while the other pulls the skin toward you, from the other side of the back. Be sure not to apply any pressure directly onto the spine as you cross over it.

Your hands should be beside each other—close enough to touch—as they move in opposite directions back and forth across the muscles. If you are wringing with the correct technique, you can see the skin and tissues underneath your hands torqueing. Work up and down the whole length of the back. You will find you can move the skin and underlying muscles quite easily. It looks awful, but feels wonderful! Be sure to check the pressure of your touch with the person on the receiving end as you massage.

This stroke is one of my patients' favorites, both pregnant and nonpregnant. There is something about the cross-fiber direction of the stroke that works on the nervous system differently from other massage strokes. It always gets the sleepiest of patients or the most relaxed moms-to-be purring and taking the effort to make a positive comment (especially at the knee, a favorite spot for wringing).

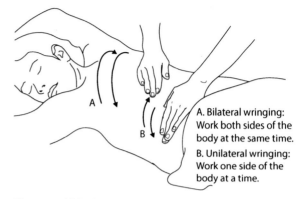

A. Bilateral wringing: Work both sides of the body at the same time.
B. Unilateral wringing: Work one side of the body at a time.

Figure 1.5. Wringing.

For the knee, I use a whole-handed wringing with an open hand above and below the kneecap housing the patella in between—a favorite with all my patients. Although you most often use your whole palmar surface for wringing, you can also use your thumbs for smaller areas, such as around the knees or on the ankles. I use thumb wringing at the base of the knee, at the attachment of the quadriceps tendon to the lower leg, and also at the ankle, wringing the front of the ankle joint when the mom is supine, or at the Achilles tendon attachment when she's prone.

This stroke can be never overused. It is like the effleurage stroke that I use in between other strokes. It comes in really handy when someone is unable to turn or be arranged face down. The mom can be in a face-up position and get the backs of her legs massaged with a thorough wrap-around wringing.

Kneading

Kneading strokes involve the alternate squeezing and relaxing of tissues like a cat kneading your lap with its paws, alternately applying and releasing pressure. Kneading helps stimulate circulation and in turn promotes the natural healing of injuries, tears, and strains by bringing fresh blood to damaged tissue.

There is a variety of kneading strokes to use with maternity massages that ranges from big strokes using the entire palmar surface of your hand to nitpicky strokes using just the thumbs or fingertips. Sometimes you might put one hand beside the other and move them in the same direction, alternately pushing the muscle and then releasing it, usually in a semicircular direction. Other times, you might use one hand to knead while the other hand rests on or supports the mom's body. Some of my most common kneading strokes are discussed briefly in this section.

REINFORCED PALMAR KNEADING

Reinforced palmar kneading is when you put one hand on top of the other and make kneading circles. This helps you put the full weight of your body into your strokes to really focus in on tight spots in large muscles, such as the hip or back. On the back, the direction of pressure should always be up and away from the spine. On the legs or other extremities, the pressure always goes toward the heart.

In my classes, I often see how the name of the stroke causes people to use only the palm of the hand, sometimes keeping their fingers off the skin and just polishing with the heel of their hand. However, the idea for palmar kneading is more of a cupping, all-inclusive posture for the hands. Give as much skin-on-skin contact as possible with the whole palmar surface of the hand, right to the tips of the fingers.

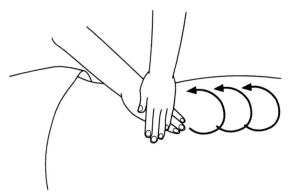

Figure 1.6. Reinforced palmar kneading (both hands, stacked).

OVERHANDED PALMAR KNEADING

Overhanded palmar kneading is another stroke I use often, especially on the abdomen or hips in side-lying posture. It is a circular stroke in which one hand chases the other around in circles, with one hand hopping over the other. Keep the right hand on the skin, doing a big circle around the abdomen around the baby. Follow your right hand with your left. When your left hand catches up to the right, hop your left hand over the right and continue around the circle. This continuous stroke is very thorough and effective for helping with digestive functioning. I also use it at the head of the femur when I am massaging the hip in side-lying positions. I often change back and forth between reinforced palmar kneading and over-handed palmar kneading for both the abdominal and hip massages.

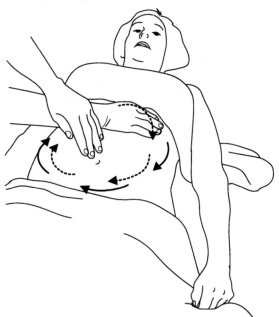

Figure 1.7. Overhanded palmar kneading. Travel around the perimeter of the abdomen and be gentle so you don't disturb the baby.

ALTERNATE THUMB KNEADING

The thumbs and fingers are also excellent instruments for kneading strokes, especially in areas of the body needing focused attention. In alternate thumb kneading, the whole hand (including fingertips) makes contact with the skin, but the thumbs do the work. First one thumb and then the other makes small half to three-quarter overlapping circles over the skin. If your thumbs get tired, give your hands a good shake to loosen them up.

You want your thumbs balanced in their alternating rotations, pushing up and out along the direction of the muscle fibers, always with the pressure of each circle going up to the heart. I encourage my students to talk out loud to get their thumbs into a rhythm, saying "up and out . . . up and out . . . up and out . . . right and left . . . right and left . . . right and left . . . up and out . . . ." I learned early on in my teaching that there is something about saying something three times that glues it into the brain the right way. I often take my students for a ride on my thumbs so they can feel the momentum and balance of alternate thumb kneading.

Years ago, my students usually found that the thumb on their dominant hand would know what to do, but their other thumb would be clumsy and unable to accomplish full circles. Today, I find a shift as people are becoming naturally ambidextrous because of the use of electronic communication devices. Flying left thumbs are becoming a thing of the past.

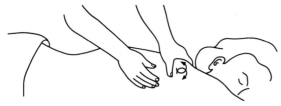

Figure 1.8. Alternate thumb kneading.

This is the stroke I use in my maternity massages to deal with the most painful places. Use this stroke on the attachments of muscles, in the bulk of muscles, and in any knots or tight spots. I use this stroke after general strokes to the iliotibial band, head of the femur, or any other structures at the top of the leg. I find that the tiny focus of this stroke really works to ease tension in muscles. The back and forth of the overlapping strokes has both a calming and stimulating influence.

In the first trimester, this stroke is the staple of my massage routine. I use alternate thumb kneading everywhere, especially on the legs and arms. Probably the only place I don't use it is on the face. The stroke is particularly appreciated in the extremities, at the inner elbow and inner forearm, and around the knees and ankles, which are ideal spots to do long sessions of alternate thumb kneading.

Alternate thumb kneading always gets lots of calls for encores. This stroke is wonderfully designed to treat prenatal aches and pains. Simply repeatedly going over an area that is sore with your alternating thumbs will slowly and steadily relax the tissues.

Move back and forth between alternate thumb kneading and the more general strokes of palmar kneading or wringing. Don't wear out your welcome with too much alternate thumb kneading! Use general strokes to smooth things out, effectively erasing the discomfort, and then you can go back again to do another set of thumb kneading.

Single-handed thumb kneading is useful when you need to secure the mom with one hand. In my latest delivery, I used one hand to hold on to the side of the mom's hip and used the other hand to work away at the spasms in her hip muscles. I kneaded with a circular movement of my thumb to the muscle and then I switched hands and did the same with the other hand. One hand secured the hip and the other hand did the massaging.

FINGERTIP KNEADING

Fingertips can also be used to knead, usually with reinforced fingertip kneading. Stack your hands on top of each other and keep your fingers straight and stiff. Then knead with a pivoting action of your wrist so your fingertips are like a soft drill. As with thumbs, you can also knead with one hand if you need to stabilize the mom's body with your other hand.

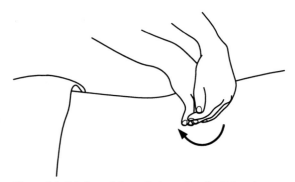

Figure 1.9. Reinforced fingertip kneading (both hands, fingers stacked).

Thumb stretching

SHORT STROKES

Thumb stretching is a little like alternate thumb kneading, but instead of the thumbs moving in overlapping circles, the thumb tips or sides move in overlapping straight strokes of steady pressure to stretch out the tissue underneath. Push your alternating thumbs ahead and away from you, so they are like a combination Ferris wheel and conveyor belt. Start with the thumb pads and move to the thumb tips for greater focus, pokiness, depth, and precision. This is also a transverse stroke that can be performed using the side of the thumbs—not the tips—across the erector spinae muscles.

LONG STROKES

You can also do this type of thumb stretching with long, continuous strokes. On the back, use a long, continuous movement of the tips of your thumbs in the groove between the spine and erector spinae muscles. Move your thumbs slowly—very slowly all the way up this groove. You can never be too slow! Moving slowly may help you find where muscles are bunched up, indicating a place to be worked on. I sometimes alternate this stroke with short, overlapping thumb stretching strokes in the same groove or right on top of the erector spinae.

Scooping

Scooping is often done with a closed-fingered, cupped hand like you would use to scoop a handful of water. I use this stroke on the neck, scooping up toward the head, or on the shoulders with my patient lying supine, scooping from the bottom of the shoulder blades up the neck in an alternating scooping style.

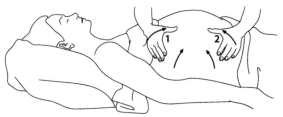

Figure 1.10. Scooping can also be done with a wide open, C-shaped hand. Alternate between your hands as you scoop.

In maternity massage, I use scooping primarily with breast massage. The scooping of the breasts is performed with an alternating movement between the two hands. It is an upward milking stroke with the hands scooping the breast in a lifting motion. It is as though each hand passes the breast off to the other hand in an alternating action.

Tapotement

Tapotement is a percussive movement. In pregnancy, it is used for stress relief and the encouragement of deep relaxation. Although I don't use it often in a regular pregnancy massage, I always use it in labor and delivery.

Tapotement strokes are also part of my "care for the caregivers" lesson for head, neck, and shoulder massages in my classes for pregnant couples. I always get caregivers to sit on the floor between the knees of their pregnant partner so she can practice on their shoulders and upper back. A regular application of these tapotement strokes will keep their partners working well during labor and delivery. In my last delivery, I used more pounding on the dad's back than the mom's as Darren really benefited from the relief this stroke produced for his low back.

LOOSE FINGERTIP HACKING

This stroke is great for the upper shoulders and is done for someone laboring sitting up if her arms and shoulders ache from holding her legs or knees up in active pushing. Take both hands and put them in a prayer position close to each other. Alternate lifting each hand and striking the surface in a hacking motion. Your fingers should be loose, so your fingertips will flick against each other. Only the little finger side of the hand will make contact with the person on the receiving end of this invigorating stroke. (Figure 1.11a)

Once you get a rhythm, speed it up so your hands are a blur of activity. The trick is to keep your hands from tangling up with each other. Most people find that one hand will keep a steady rhythm while the other will be all over the place. But the more you practice, the better you will get at keeping your hands balanced and even in tempo and strength.

Shake out your hands when your hacking gets lopsided or your hands get tangled up. The shake will help you reset.

STIFF FINGERTIP HACKING

This stroke is similar to loose fingertip hacking, but you keep your fingertips together, glued to each other. The action of the hand lifting up and down is more controlled. The fingers do not flick against each other, but rather hold tight to each other in a chopping motion. (Figure 1.11b)

Both hacking strokes are used on the upper shoulders and the entire back in either a face-down position or side-lying. Side-lying is more awkward and the person doing the massage is going to have to adapt by raising the hospital bed or squatting down to angle the hands properly to massage the spinal muscles running up and down the back (the erector spinae). Be sure to balance strokes on both sides of the body. If the mom can turn over, you can do the stroke twice.

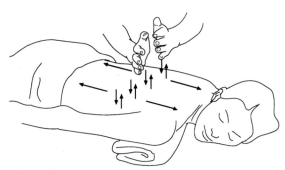

a. Loose fingertip hacking

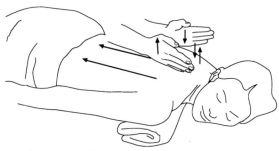

b. Stiff fingertip hacking

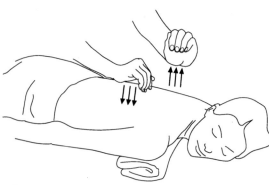

c. Cupping

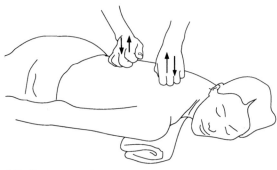

d. Beating

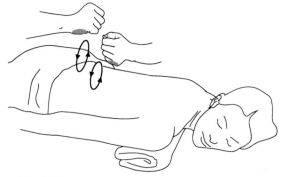

e. Pounding

Figure 1.11. Tapotement strokes. I don't use much tapotement in my regular maternity massages, but I always use them in labor and delivery. Keep your tapotement strokes on the front or back of the body, not the sides. The exception is cupping, which works nicely along the angle of the ribs at the side of the body to treat respiratory conditions.

CUPPING

This is a favorite tapotement stroke. Cup your hands and bring them down in a fairly fast drum beat, which should create a hollow sound. The most common mistake students make is keeping their fingers straight, so be sure to keep the curve of your palm extending all the way out to your fingertips. If the sound is not hollow or your partner says the stroke stings, cup your hands more. When you soften the stroke by cupping your hands properly, you will hear the difference immediately. The slapping sound will turn into a hollow sound. (Figure 1.11c)

Cupping is a traditional treatment of the respiratory conditions, such as shortness of breath, congestion, or coughs and chest colds. The stroke helps to dislodge congestion in the lungs and aids in expectoration. Cupping is usually done only on the back and the ribs. In side-lying, you can apply cupping to the upper aspect of the ribs, which is more accessible in this position than in any other.

BEATING

Beating sounds terrible but feels wonderful. Tuck your thumbs into your hands to make a fist. Then flatten out the fist into a monkey paw. Use the knuckled surface of the hand in a palms-down posture to make contact with the person's skin. The hands alternate up and down with loose wrists. (Figure 1.11d and Figure 1.12)

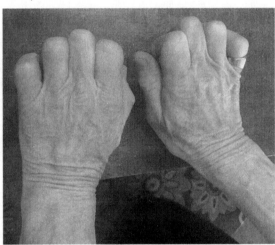

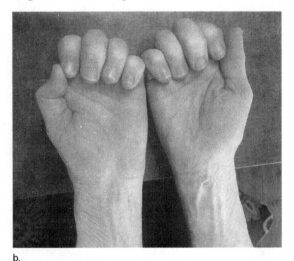

a.

b.

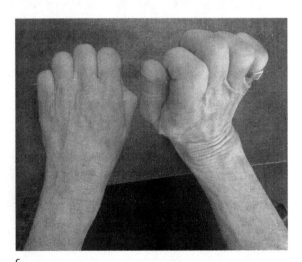

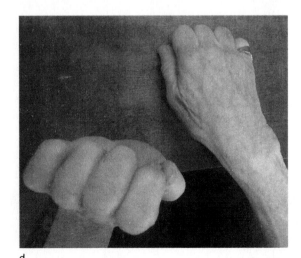

c.

d.

Figure 1.12. Beating is a movement of the hands up and down from the wrists, not the whole arms.

POUNDING

Pounding is a labor and delivery favorite! This stroke, when applied to the low back and sacrum, will expand the woman's tolerance for back labor. This stroke is like local anesthetic as it numbs the area that is feeling the contraction, usually the low back. I use a rolling pounding style of tapotement on the sacrum for this purpose. This rolling tapotement is the same stroke I use when mountain climbing to relieve low back tension from backpacks or prolonged hiking. About one minute of rolling tapotement on the low back will erase the achiness of the hike and freshen the low back for another few hours of hard work.

Make tight fists, thumbs tucked in. This makes a cushion on the ulnar border (little finger side) of the hand that makes contact. A tight fist has a softer impact than if the hand is loose, which can feel like a bony surface. You don't want the stroke rebounding off the back; instead, use a rolling application where the fists make a circular movement between impacts. The result is a sort of pounding caress. (Figure 1.11e)

The pounding can be done when the laboring mom is seated, lying on her side, or on her hands and knees in delivery mode. Use it on top of towels and clothing; it doesn't need to be skin to skin. You can even do the rolling pounding on top of a soft ice pack that conform to the body's shape.

Frictioning

Frictioning is a highly therapeutic cross-fiber stroke used to wear down adhesions, which are areas of tissue that build up in response to injuries, infection, or postsurgical conditions. Tears or other injuries in the belly of muscles or their attachments to ligaments and other structures are healed by a glue-like substance called fibrin. Fibrin adhesions are inelastic, which can limit normal function, movement, and flexibility. Adhesions can even cause infertility, endometriosis, and other internal organ malfunctions and discomforts. Frictioning can break down adhesions and improve elasticity in muscles and ligaments. If it is done properly, frictioning can lead to decreased pain and increased function.

Frictioning is usually performed by professionals with a strong knowledge of gross anatomy, but I have been able to help many people by teaching their families how to use this therapeutic technique. The mom can even use frictioning as part of a self-massage.

I use frictioning a lot with my athletic pregnant patients who have old injuries from childhood or adolescent sports that limit their hip mobility for easy deliveries. Sometimes the mom can tell you where she's had an injury or has tight spots. You can feel the adhesion area as a thickening in the muscle. The mom will give you feedback when you've found the right place. She'll likely feel some discomfort when you press on it.

Put your fingertips together. I usually use my pointer and middle fingers, but sometimes I use my thumb. Use the tips of your fingers to find the site of an adhesion. Once the mom confirms you're at the right place, start to rub your fingertips back and forth quickly, as though you are erasing the spot of the adhesion. Use pressure, but check in with the mom frequently to be sure she can tolerate the stroke. I alternate the frictioning with a knuckled effleurage to smooth out the friction site and then I apply the frictioning again.

You are basically working to soften and stretch the tough adhesion under your fingers. You will have to use pressure to get this result but, as always, ask the mom whether your pressure is too much, not enough, or just right. Usually if you have the right location, the mom will find the stroke uncomfortable, but tolerable. Remember that this is in the middle of your treatment, not the beginning. Other strokes will have "primed" it for this focused and sometimes uncomfortable treatment.

I often use ice as a frictioning tool for the anesthetizing effect of the cold as my fingers soften and break down the hard fibers. In my latest delivery, the mom insisted we keep frictioning and kneading her gluteals to lessen their muscle spasms.

Vibrations

Vibrations have a fast, shaky quality, like getting "nervous" with your hand. Using bent or straight arms, produce fine, trembling vibrations with your palms or fingertips. Stiffen up the arms and then finely bounce up and down on the skin or make a side-to-side vibratory movement. Palmar vibrations can be made with the palms stacked (reinforced) or side by side. Fingertip movements can be static (in one place) or running (moving from one spot to another).

Vibrations are useful for respiratory or digestive blockages. Very light, fluttering types of vibrations can work along nerve routes for neurological soothing. Most North American massage therapists use electronic vibrations, but European massage therapists often use a bent elbow or stiff, straight arm as the way to apply the stroke.

In my early instruction, I was taught not to apply pressure with this stroke, but I use firm pressure, copying my experiences being on the receiving-end of vibrations in Germany. My massage therapist, a Roman Catholic nun wearing a full black and white habit, drilled away with running and static vibrations with a huge tremor quality. I had a deep relaxation response, sleeping two rejuvenating hours.

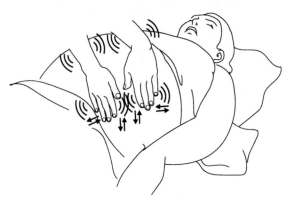

Figure 1.13. Vibrations can be with a fine side-to-side or up-and-down movement.

Light reflex stroking

A good finishing stroke is light reflex stroking, which is moving your hands with a light touch over the body. On the back, simultaneously glide your fingers along each side of the spine from the neck down to the low back. Then switch to overhanded stroking, with your hands moving like a conveyor belt of continuous sensation as one hand lifts off

at the low back and the other hand makes contact at the neck. Then switch back to both hands at once, but whatever combination you do, keep the flow going for five or six strokes. Make each time lighter or slower than the last so you finish with your hands hovering over the person's skin.

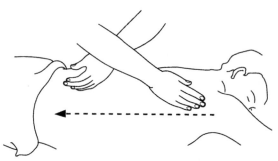

Figure 1.14. Light reflex stroking is a nice finish to massage. For butterfly stroking, add a flicker movement to your fingertips.

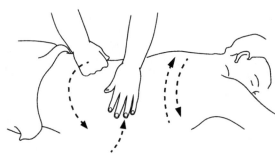

Figure 1.15. A variation of reflex stroking is a modified form of wringing. This variation uses the back of your fingers for the stroke away and then the palmar side of your fingers as you move toward you. When stroking away, start with the first knuckles of your fingers and then gradually move to the middle digits and then the fingertips.

The Finale

For all massage routines in this book, try to back out of the massage the same way you went in. The three strokes of effleurage, wringing, and reinforced palmar kneading are used as the final book end when I am finished with the more focused massage strokes that make up the middle of any massage sequence. I start with these three strokes and usually end with the same three strokes.

All you need to do is remember to always finish by smoothing out the stirred-up sensations where you have focused your treatment with wringing and reinforced palmar kneading and finally, effleurage. Then the patient does not have my trigger points, frictioning, or any of my other thumbprints talking to her the next day. Light reflex stroking is a nice finish if you're ending the massage or moving to a new body part. You want to make sure the person (like the horse in the barn) is looking forward to having another body part massaged! As always, a soak in a relaxing Epsom salt bath makes a postmassage mediative moment.

Positioning

First-trimester massages can be done in traditional positions for nonpregnant women (face down or face up). After four or five months, the side-lying posture is a classic and traditional treatment posture. You can also use the side-lying position in the first trimester if the mom has had lower-back issues or sciatica before pregnancy. This position will avoid causing any increased strain on her low back during the massage.

Supine (face-up) positioning

Place pillows under the knees and under the head to flex the head slightly up for better breathing. If the mom has leg swelling, you might use extra pillows to elevate her legs for drainage. If she's having trouble breathing, use more pillows behind her back and head to create a slightly sitting position. By the third trimester, you might have to support her with enough pillows to sit almost upright so she can breathe. Before you start, place a hot water bottle, hot pack, or warm microwave beanbag under the mom's neck and feet.

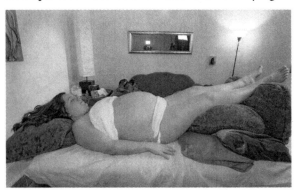

Figure 1.16. Jessica, a maternity nurse with a fourth pregnancy, here shows supine lying with lots of pillow support.

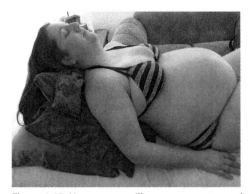

Figure 1.17. Use as many pillows as necessary to elevate the mom's head so she can breathe easier.

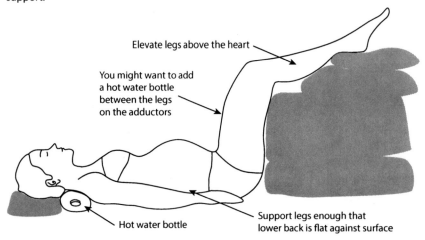

Elevate legs above the heart

You might want to add a hot water bottle between the legs on the adductors

Hot water bottle

Support legs enough that lower back is flat against surface

Figure 1.18. Keys to comfortable supine positioning in pregnancy.

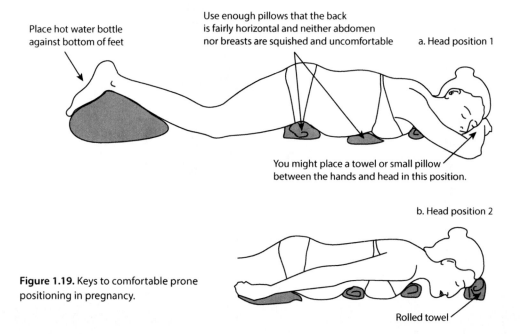

Place hot water bottle against bottom of feet

Use enough pillows that the back is fairly horizontal and neither abdomen nor breasts are squished and uncomfortable

a. Head position 1

You might place a towel or small pillow between the hands and head in this position.

b. Head position 2

Figure 1.19. Keys to comfortable prone positioning in pregnancy.

Rolled towel

Prone (face-down) positioning

Use a rolled towel for the upper chest above the breasts, supporting the sternum and taking pressure off the breasts. The towel needs to be long enough to curl around under the armpits. This support will also help the mom extend and turn her neck without discomfort. If she wants, she can rest her head on stacked hands or another rolled towel under her forehead.

Use two pillows under the mom's ankles to semiflex the legs and take pressure off the low back. Women who have a bit of a sway back may need extra support for the low back. I also position pillows to support the abdominal area, giving the back a more even and horizontal line. Place a hot water bottle on the mom's feet.

Whether face down or face up, having the legs in a semiflexed position will relieve pressure on the low back. Anyone with a lower-back problem will be able to tell you how effective this simple technique is for making lying down comfortable. With this support, you can press on the mom's back and not cause any discomfort for the vertebrae.

The face-down position may seem impossible for the third trimester, but with proper pillow support, you should be able to keep the mom comfortable right to the end of her pregnancy. Use as many pillows as needed under the hips to avoid pressure on the baby. Balance this with more support between the breasts and baby with rolled towels so no one gets squished! Also place pillows under the mom's ankles to semiflex her legs and ease the pull or strain on her low back.

With this support, the mom should be comfortable for at least thirty minutes. This is great for people with bad backs if the only way to find relief is through massage in a face-down resting position. Years ago, I learned from my pregnant patients how to do this pillow positioning and today it still works wonders!

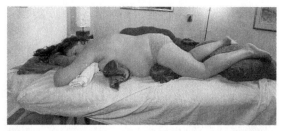

Figure 1.20. With the right pillow support, even a mom in her third trimester can lie comfortably on her front.

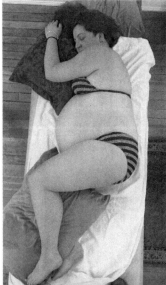

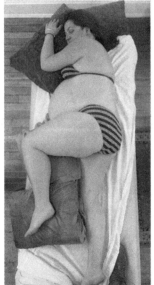

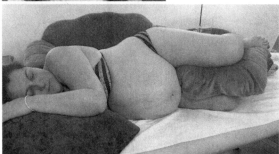

Figure 1.21. Full-crooked patient position.

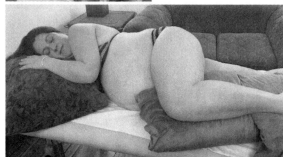

Figure 1.22. Half-crooked patient position.

Side-lying position

Side-lying is used in the second and third trimesters and is also indicated for the first trimester if the mom has issues in the low back, sacroiliac strain, sciatica, or any other back problem.

Use pillows to keep the mom in position so she doesn't roll onto her front as you push on her back. You will also want to use pillow support to keep her hips from twisting and to keep her back in a flat, untwisted plane. Use a pillow under her head to keep it up, not angled downward. This will help her breathing so she doesn't get stuffed up.

FULL-CROOKED PATIENT POSITIONING

This means the mom is in a curled fetal position, with chin tucked slightly toward the chest and both knees bent up together at a ninety-degree angle. I find this position best so I can lean on the mom's back without rolling her onto her front. Place pillows between her knees to bring the top knee height up so the leg is horizontal and not angled downward. (Figure 1.21)

HALF-CROOKED PATIENT POSITIONING

This means the upper knee is bent up and the bottom leg is straight. Place a pillow under the top knee to keep the hip from twisting. I have found that this position is good for lots of women in resting, but in side-lying for massage, this posture has more tendency to have the woman roll forward when you exert massage pressure on her back.

Tucking the mom's head down so her chin is toward her chest puts her into a more curled and fetal position. Place a pillow under the head, angled toward the front between the breasts. Most people instinctively push the pillow back from the front of them to over their shoulder. I bring it back down around to the front and instruct them to put one hand under and the other hand on top of the pillow. (Figure 1.22)

I use the full-crooked position most of the time, but I'll use whatever is the most comfortable position for the mom whether I am massaging her in her pregnancy or labor.

Draping Protocols

Draping helps keep your patient relaxed and not worried about exposing her private parts, especially when friends and extended family are part of the massage team. But aside from questions of modesty, proper draping is important to help the patient conserve the heat generated by the massage. The heat helps the relaxation response, so you want to retain as much of it as possible.

Use big towels or a sheet to cover parts of the body that aren't being worked on. For example, while massaging the abdomen, use a towel to cover the breasts. Tuck the ends of the towel under the armpits or over the shoulders. When massaging the legs, use towels or a sheet to cover the mom's torso and arms.

I always tuck the sheeting firmly up against the mom so she can feel its pressure. Draping for side-lying may take some practice, but the mom can usually help you tuck in the ends of the towel or sheet.

Massage Postures for the Massager

As part of the maternity team, you, as the massager, need to keep healthy and strong. Be sure to protect your back from strain, or you won't be of any help later in the pregnancy. In general, your position should be comfortable, sustainable, and using the least amount of energy for maximum efficiency. The following tips should help you avoid strains or injuries:

- Wear comfortable shoes and clothing.
- If the mom is lying on a table, have her lie near the edge so she is close to your body. This will help you keep your back upright.

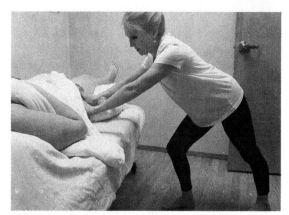
Figure 1.23. The leg in front should be closest to the person you're massaging.

- Keep your knees bent, with one leg in front of the other to execute a smooth rocking motion with as little effort as possible (stride posture).
- When effleuraging the entire leg, take a step or two alongside the table at the same time as the arm movement to prevent overreaching.
- If you're working on the floor, take a shiatsu position, with one knee on the floor and one knee up. The knee on the floor should be closest to the mom. Use your legs to get a forward rocking motion.

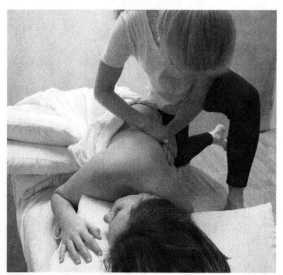
Figure 1.24. The shiatsu position provides good back support if you're working on the floor or the bed beside the mom.

- When the mom is in a seated position, take a stride position with one foot ahead of the other so you can lean forward without straining your back.

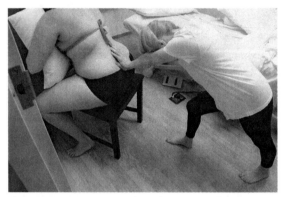

Figure 1.25. Lean in to get the right amount of pressure, but be sure your legs take the stride position. This position is excellent for pain management during labor!

Learn how to position yourself comfortably and safely. This is the key to stamina so you don't give in to awkward postures that can hurt your back.

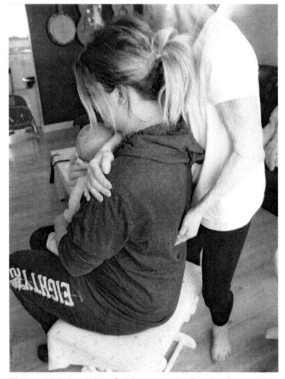

Figure 1.26. Don't be afraid to move in close to the mom. In this position, brace her with one arm and use the other to work on her back.

Ending the Massage

All your work will generate a lot of warmth in the mom's body. Take advantage of this warmth by covering her up and allowing her some time to just lie still. She may find this an excellent time for meditation, prayer, or visualization. She can use the massage as a vehicle for deeper experiences of letting go. An Epsom salt bath (described on page 12) can deepen the relaxation effects of the massage and help her get more mileage out of your massage.

End the massage by washing your hands and then rinsing with cool water, which will help ground you and cut down on the possibility of energy transference from the person you're massaging to yourself.

KNEIPP HYDROTHERAPY

My routine of rinsing my hands with cold water is one aspect of Kneipp therapy that I learned in Bad Wörishofen, Germany, which I visited in 1984 to see if they would let me bring their Kneipp hydrotherapy to Canada. In the nineteenth century, Sebastian Kneipp, a Catholic priest and naturopath, developed the practice of using cold water (and sometimes alternating warm and cold water) as a therapy for various ailments. He became famous for his "water cure" after curing his own tuberculosis with cold water from the Danube River. He went on to research cold water applications to promote health and to treat patients with various diseases.

The rationale for cold water treatments lies in how well a cold application helps stimulate the body's circulation, which in turn promotes healing. With the shock of cold on the skin, the blood vessels immediately constrict (vasoconstriction). Then there is a secondary response—vasodilation—as the body sends blood rushing to the area, creating warmth and a reddening color. It is as if the body, to fight the cold, decides to send in the (circulatory) troops to warm things up as quickly as possible.

It's easier to stimulate circulation with cold than with heat alone. The body is already warm at 98.6°F, so you can't heat it up much more without burning or causing other damage to the tissues. However, if you reduce the temperature with cold, you have a greater temperature range to warm the tissues without causing damage.

Kneipp's treatments are today used by many medical professionals; massage therapists often find it a wonderful enhancement of their work. Hydrotherapy, the use of water to treat various conditions, is a big part of my massage practice. I use cold water and ice as a way to speed up the body's natural healing processes. I also use a small bucket of cold water and some witch hazel to wash each body part after I massage it. In an adaptation of Kneipp's techniques, I use ice massage as a pain remedy and to treat everything from surgical incisions to adhesions around wound sites. Ice massage stimulates the cells around the perimeter of wounds or ulcer sites to accelerate cell renewal.

In chapter 6, I describe uses of hydrotherapy for breast health in pregnant and nursing women. Another favorite use of hydrotherapy for pregnant or postpartum women is the cold water contrast footbath to encourage circulation, reduce swelling, and alleviate headaches.

COLD WATER CONTRAST FOOTBATH

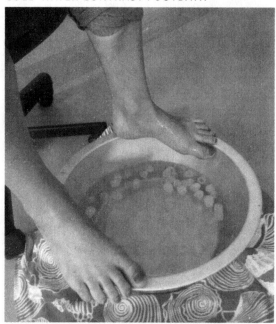

Figure 1.27. An ice water footbath is good for both swollen feet and headaches.

1. Soak your feet for five minutes in a bucket of warm water (approximately 36°C, 97°F).
2. Move your feet for ten seconds to a bucket of cold water (approximately 18°C, 65°F).
3. Remove your feet from the cold water for ten seconds.
4. Repeat steps 2 and 3 ten times, and then dry your feet.
5. Put on warm socks or move around to warm the feet again.

Massage Treatments for the Trimesters

Massage is important for every stage of maternity, from before conception, through the pregnancy trimesters, and into the postnatal period, what I sometimes call the "fourth trimester." There is never too much massage for these transitions of life.

I tend to do the full maternity massage, including tummy, with every prenatal patient in my practice, but I adjust my proportions of how much time each body part gets based on what my patient wants or needs. I always ask the woman what she is most looking forward to for the massage I'm about to give and I ask her what she benefited most from after her last massage treatment. After positioning the woman comfortably with pillows, I apply hot packs under the neck and feet and then quickly do a "once-over" on the extremities before I go back to any areas of focus.

Self-massage

Self-massage techniques are useful for every stage of pregnancy. Bath time is often a good opportunity for self-massage, but the mom can work self-massage into other times of the day, too. I encourage my pregnant patients to roll golf or tennis balls under their rear ends whenever sitting (at work, in the car, while watching television, etc.) This will help keep the gluteals supple, an investment in keeping everything elastic for the baby's arrival. The balls can also be used while seated to massage tight spots in the back.

In the third trimester, the mom can help work to open her inner thighs with self-massage to the adductors. Self-massage is also a critical part of breast care during the pregnancy and postpartum. Details on breast massage are in chapter 6.

Schedule

Most professional massages run about one hour in length, but home massages do not need to be as long. The most important thing is frequency, so aim for daily massages, even if each is only twenty or thirty minutes.

In preparation for the birth of the baby, it is great to have a schedule for massages by family and friends, a professional, or both. Although I recommend as many massages as possible, I also know people have work and other family obligations. The following outline gives suggestions for a minimum number of massages for each trimester, but if you can do more, all the better! The more massage the mom receives, the better she will thrive throughout her pregnancy and delivery.

- **First trimester**: In the first trimester, I recommend a full-body massage every week to get the pregnancy off to a great start and for bonding and energy input by the dad or partner. Friends factor into this scenario if you build your birthing team beyond intimate family members. I recommend a professional massage at least every second week.

- **Second trimester**: In the second trimester, I recommend a professional full-body massage once a week, with the other family massages as often as possible on a daily basis. Foot massages take a special focus here as the mom's feet get bigger and puffier as the weight upon them increases. Back symptoms begin to show up as the spine is pulled forward with the growing baby, increasing the lower-back lordotic curve. Side-lying postures are now used to treat sacroiliac strain, sciatica, and hip problems.

- **Third trimester**: In the third trimester, the massages can never be too many! I suggest the couples massage thoroughly once a week for the first month of the last trimester and then double it up each month that follows. So the second-to-last month is twice a week at home with partners and the last month is three times a week, basically every other day. This schedule reduces stress and is engaging for the dad or birth partner. It keeps everyone busy and not feeling helpless about the growing discomforts of pregnancy.

It's great if everyone on the birthing team can take turns doing the full-body massages this last month. I have some patients I see every day in the last two weeks of their term because they cannot manage without daily massage for breathing, sleeping, eating, and moving. The excitement of "false" or warm-up labor will give you a chance to practice labor and delivery massage techniques for the contractions.

- **Imminent delivery**: Imminent delivery (starting one week before the due date) should prompt daily massage until the delivery. Your massages will now focus on the areas of direct labor and delivery significance, such as the inner thighs and the perineal floor of the pelvis. This lead-up to delivery will accustom the birthing team to all the massage routines and techniques to use in hospital or home births. These "waiting" massages are great stress relievers for everyone, especially if waiting for an overdue baby.

First Trimester Massage

The most common symptoms at this stage are nausea, breast enlargement, dietary peculiarities, and extremes of emotions. First-time moms or moms who have had miscarriages or trouble conceiving may naturally feel anxious. Other physical symptoms resulting from the baby's growth (trouble breathing, swollen feet, etc.) are not usually troublesome at this point. Because of this, in the first trimester, I generally use my basic full-body massage (for nonpregnant people), supplemented with a breast massage and/or an abdominal or diaphragmatic massage, which is helpful for nausea. However, every pregnancy is different, so you may need to dip into techniques from the second and third trimesters, or those listed for specific symptoms in chapter 3.

My basic massage sequence outlined here is a guideline to get you started. Other than starting and finishing with effleurage and wringing, the rest is up to you and the mom you're massaging. Ask her what she wants or needs! No two women have the same pregnancy, so no two will want or need the same massage. For example, the focus for my patient Nadine at eight weeks was nausea. She wanted abdominal massages and a headache treatment with lots of time spent on the head, neck, and shoulders. Another first-trimester patient, Sheila, wanted her breasts to be a focus of our massages, as she was bursting out of her clothing and her breasts were heavy and hot. I used a combination of hydrotherapy and massage on both these different first-trimester pregnancies.

In general, touching firmly and continuously is the best soother of a nervous system charged up with all the changes going on in the body during the first trimester of pregnancy.

Timing

First trimester massages should be at least once a week. Make it a special time with candles and great food before or after. Use the following timetable for the first trimester, which will allow you to deliver your massage in an hour:

- Five minutes for each leg and arm, face up or face down
- Five minutes for the face and scalp
- Twenty minutes for the back, face down or side-lying
- Fifteen minutes for the front

You might want to add in five minutes of massage for an area of concern, such as the forearms if the mom works in an office or is on a computer a lot, or do extra massage for the low back or legs. You can add to or otherwise revise this basic timeline as you progress in your skills and as the mom's needs grow.

Patient positioning

Most of the time, you can massage a woman in the first trimester like you would massage a nonpregnant person, using face up, face down, or side-lying—whatever is most comfortable for her. Refer to pages 26–29 for proper pillow support in all positioning.

Massage for the first trimester

BACK

Face-down back massage is normal in the first trimester because the baby is not yet pulling at the mom's low back. Do each stroke in the sequence three times or more.

1. **Effleurage**: Starting at the low back or shoulders, head up or down the erector spinae muscles that run parallel to the spine, about an inch away from the spine on both sides. When you reach the neck or low back, circle to the outside edges of the back and pull toward you. On the back you can use equal pressure on your strokes while pushing away from you along the erector spinae muscles and while pulling back toward you along the sides. Pressure both ways is fine. Ask the mom if she wants the stroke firmer.

2. **Wringing**: Starting anywhere on the back, place your hands across the long muscles of the spinal corridor. Reach across the mom's back with one hand as far as you can reach. Place the other hand on the side of the mom closest to you. Move your hands toward each

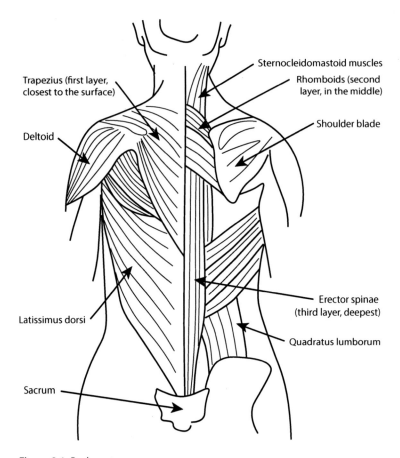

Figure 2.1. Back anatomy.

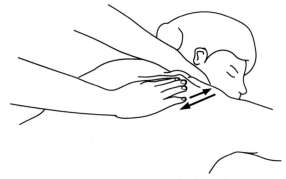

Figure 2.2. Don't miss wringing the shoulders. Scrumple the skin between your wringing hands to provide a delicious sensation for the mom.

other, with a grip firm enough to move the skin and tissue underneath. As your hands pass closely by each other in the middle of the back, they will be wringing the skin between them. (Figures 1.5 and 2.2)

3. **Kneading**: Use alternate thumb kneading up and down the erector spinae muscles. The strokes move in the direction of the muscle fibers. After the erector spinae, I do further kneading anywhere the mom wants me to go. Between the shoulder blades and spine is a favorite spot for many women. I might alternate between various forms of kneading: palmar, reinforced fingertip, and thumbs, with the understanding that the thumbs and fingers give more direct, focused attention (and potentially more therapeutic effect). Don't jump right into the most uncomfortable strokes. If you focus on an area with these direct strokes, back off once in a while with a couple of wringing or effleurage strokes. Then you can go back in again with more focused work. If the mom has any old injuries, add in some frictioning.

My "go-to" places for back massage kneading include the following:

- low back
- sacrum
- the attachments of the back to the upper edge of the pelvis
- in the rhomboids between the shoulder blades

4. **Neck massage**: Stand at the head of the table or bed and spend time at the neck with a scooping motion to the hands. This is like what you would do for a scooping breast massage, but instead you alternate your hands as they scoop the tissue up the back of the neck to the head. Add some fingertip kneading to the base of the skull. Work any tension out of the neck with fingertip kneading to the sternocleidomastoid muscles running along the sides of the neck to the front. Add some wringing to smooth things out, and then finish with a couple of strokes that link the neck and back all together, such as wringing and effleurage.

5. **Light reflex stroking**: Finish off the back with some light reflex stroking using your fingertips. This stroke will heighten the relaxation response in a soothing fashion. It is the finishing touch before moving on to the legs.

SAMPLE BACK MASSAGE ROUTINE

1. Effleurage (3x)	5 minutes
2. Wringing (3x)	
3. Reinforced palmar kneading/ single-handed palmar kneading (3x)	10 minutes
4. Alternate thumb kneading/single-handed thumb kneading	
5. Reinforced fingertip kneading/ single-handed fingertip kneading	
6. Wringing (3x)	5 minutes
7. Effleurage (3x)	
8. Light reflex stroking (10x)	

LEGS (PRONE)

1. **Effleurage**: Do at least three effleurage strokes up and down the leg, remembering to apply pressure only on the up stroke.

On the way up the leg, lean onto your hands and push them away from you with steady pressure. Keep your hands ahead of you as they travel up the leg from the foot to the hip. You may have to walk beside the bedside or table so you do not overextend your back. The pressure must come from your whole body weight or you will just be using your arm power instead of your full-body power. Put one leg out in front of the other in a stride position, your outside leg ahead (so you will naturally lean forward onto your hands, thereby putting pressure on the mom's body). If you keep your legs together, you can't get the proper pressure.

Your hands should be side by side, wrapped across the leg, not pointing up the leg. Glue them together so they act as one force. At the top of the thigh, head to the outside of the leg at the hip so you can feel the head of the femur (that sticking-out part at the side of the thigh or hip) under your palms or the heels of your hands. (Figure 2.4)

Split your hands at the head of the femur, and slowly head back to the foot with steady contact but no pressure, hands on either side of the leg, not side by side like you did traveling up the leg. Let your hands cover the entire surface of the leg on your backstroke, with one hand coming down the inside of the leg and the other hand coming down the outside of the leg.

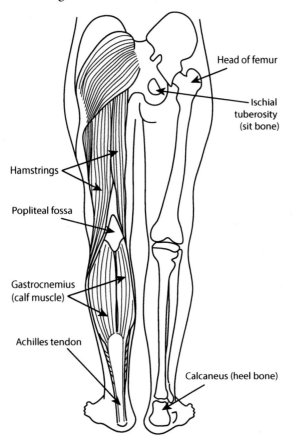

Figure 2.3. Back of leg anatomy.

On the fourth stroke up the leg, stop at the head of the femur and stay there for the next stroke of reinforced palmar kneading. This connecting stroke is like a half-effleurage.

2. **Kneading to the hip**: At the hip, massage the gluteals ("uncorking the bottle") with reinforced palmar kneading, overhanded palmar kneading, alternate thumb kneading, and then back to overhanded palmar kneading.

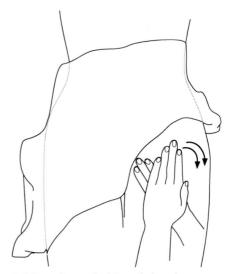

Figure 2.5. Kneading to the hip and gluteals.

3. **Hamstrings**: Apply wringing and alternate thumb kneading to the hamstrings (back of the thigh), massaging from the ischial tuberosity (the bony bump you sit on) to the popliteal fossa (back of the knee), where the tendons of the hamstring muscles attach to the lower leg. Pay extra attention to the hamstring attachments at the sides of the knee.

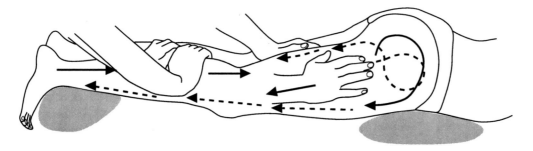

Figure 2.4. Posterior leg effleurage.

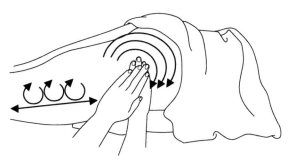

Figure 2.6. Kneading to the back of thigh and iliotibial band.

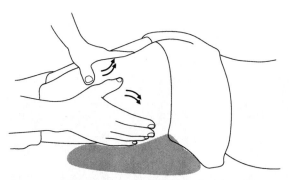

Figure 2.7. Alternate thumb kneading to the hamstrings. Move from the ischial tuberosity to the knee.

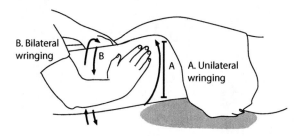

B. Bilateral wringing

B

A

A. Unilateral wringing

Figure 2.8. Wringing to the thigh offers a chance to back off some of the focused kneading strokes.

4. **Popliteal fossa:** Wring across the attachments of the gastrocnemius (calf muscle) and the hamstrings to the knee, followed by alternate thumb kneading to the entire popliteal fossa.

5. **Lower leg:** Apply wringing and alternate thumb kneading to the gastrocnemius. Give extra attention to the Achilles tendon and its attachment at the calcaneus (heel bone). In

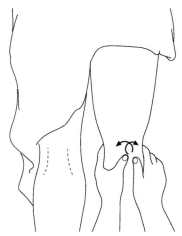

Figure 2.9. Alternate thumb kneading to the popliteal fossa.

Nelson, where there are hundreds of healthy young female athletes, this is particularly important because tendons in this town are tight. If the mom is having leg cramps, turn to page 90 to use my special "splitting the gastrocnemius" stroke, a great reliever for lower leg cramping.

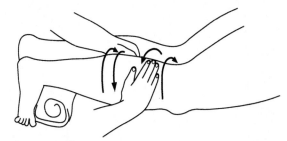

Figure 2.10. Wringing to the calf. Move from the popliteal fossa to the calcaneus.

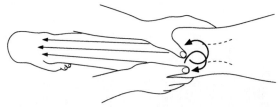

Figure 2.11. Alternate thumb kneading to the gastrocnemius. Start at the popliteal fossa and move to the heel and back again.

6. **Effleurage:** Finish with three effleurages to the full leg.

LEGS (SUPINE)

In the first trimester, you can massage the mom's legs with her lying face up or face down. With the mom face up, elevate both legs with pillows so they are higher than the heart. (This helps with postural drainage in case of any first trimester swelling in the legs.) This position also provides relief for the low back.

1. **Effleurage:** Do effleurage strokes three or four times up the leg, wrapping your hands around to the sides of the leg on the backstrokes without pressure on the way down. Use the same technique as for face-down leg massage, finishing with a half-effleurage that leaves you at the hip for a shift into reinforced palmar kneading.

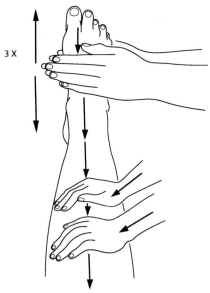

Figure 2.12. Anterior leg effleurage (3x).

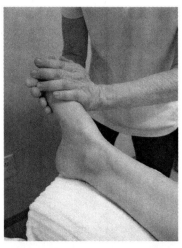

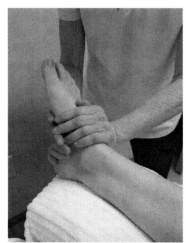

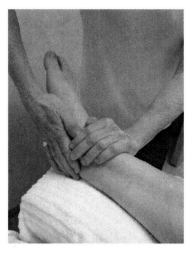

Figure 2.13. Transitioning hands from foot to leg during supine effleurage.

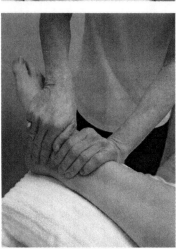

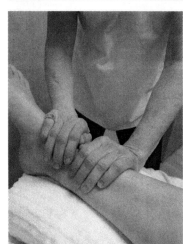

2. **Reinforced palmar kneading to the hip**:
With one hand on top of the other, begin at
the head of the femur. Here our focus is to
open up circulation between the leg and the
trunk of the body, to "uncork the bottle." All
the strokes at the top of the thigh and leg are
designed to open up the extremity to drain the
leg and also stimulate the inflow and outflow
of the lymphatics and blood.

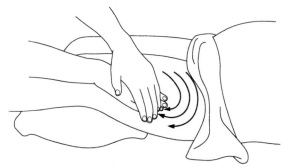

Figure 2.14. Reinforced palmar kneading to the head of the
femur.

While kneading, remember to keep the
pressure moving upward. Your hands move
in a circular direction, with a lessening of
pressure on the bottom part of the circle. I use
my body weight with this stroke, sometimes
wedging my elbows into my stomach to put
my full body weight behind my hands.

As you lean into and onto your stacked
hands, do the reinforced palmar kneading
to the head of the femur for about a minute
(which will seem like a long time); it is about
ten to twenty slow rotations of the hands.

3. **Reinforced palmar kneading to the iliotibial
band**: Move the kneading down the side of the
leg to the knee, which helps keep the iliotibial
band from tightening up and causing discomfort later on in the next trimesters. Start where
the iliotibial band attaches to the ilium (or
pelvis) and work down toward its attachment
at the tibial bump, just below the outside of the
knee. The individual pressure of each stroke
pushes up and out. Go up and down the band
about four times and then move on to other
strokes to make this structure more elastic.

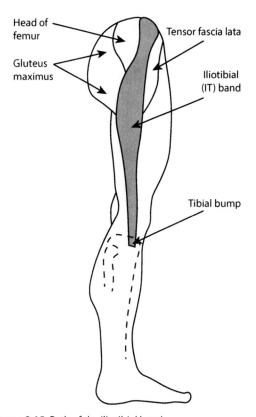

Figure 2.15. Path of the iliotibial band.

Transition: I might put a couple of effleurages
into the sequence before I go on to the thigh
wringing.

4. **Wringing to the thigh**: When wringing the
thigh, wrap your hands across the upper thigh
with a good grip, and wring right around to
the underside to include the hamstrings. The
cross-fiber stroke will help loosen the quadriceps at the front of the thighs, the hamstrings
at the back, the inner thighs (adductors), and
the iliotibial band on the outer thighs.

5. **Wringing to the iliotibial band**: The iliotibial
band is where most people hold their tension
in the lower extremities. In pregnancy, the
hormones of the first trimester start making
the pelvis more elastic, but those hormones
unfortunately don't help the iliotibial band,
although it does respond well to massage
therapy. I usually have to stand away from the
table or bed to get a good grip to wring the
outside of the thigh.

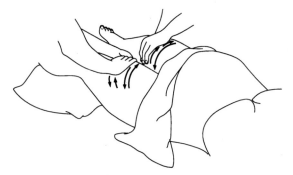

Figure 2.16. When wringing the leg, you can wring the entire leg and then focus on the upper thigh and then the knee, and then work your way down the lower leg, or you can start at the top of the leg and work your way down, saving wringing the whole leg as a finishing step.

Two areas of the leg then deserve special focus: the adductors and the knees.

6. **Adductors**: After wringing the whole leg, you may want to focus on the adductors (upper inner thigh muscles). Adductors tend to be very tight on athletic moms-to-be, but you want them to be loose and elastic in time for labor and delivery. After wringing the adductors, use alternate thumb kneading and single-handed fingertip kneading to further loosen them. Then finish with more wringing to the whole leg.

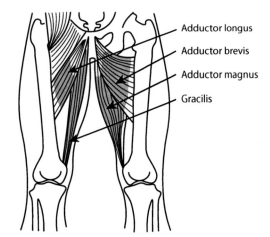

Adductor longus
Adductor brevis
Adductor magnus
Gracilis

Figure 2.17. The adductors are the muscles on the inner thigh. Massage for this area will become an increasing focus in the second and third trimesters, so it's good to begin massage on the adductors now.

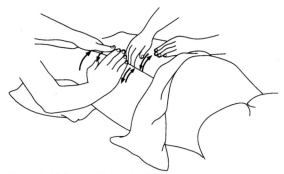

Figure 2.18. Inner thigh wringing.

7. **Wringing to the knee**: Wring around the knee and across the quadriceps. The four quadriceps muscles house the patella and insert into the common patellar tendon and then into the top of the front of the lower leg at the bump called the tibial tuberosity.

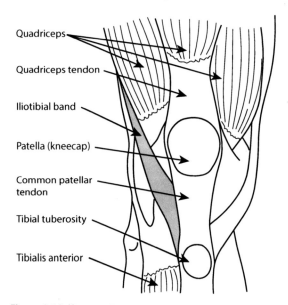

Quadriceps
Quadriceps tendon
Iliotibial band
Patella (kneecap)
Common patellar tendon
Tibial tuberosity
Tibialis anterior

Figure 2.19. Knee anatomy.

Use open palms to wring the kneecap, with one hand above the kneecap and one hand below, encasing it. Instead of the closed-hand shape used in normal wringing, use an open hand with the thumb stretched away from the other fingers. You can spend up to five minutes wringing around the knee. I also use a special cutting-style wringing in this area, using one thumb to slice across the top of the kneecap and the other thumb to slice across the bottom. The two thumbs have the kneecap wedged between them.

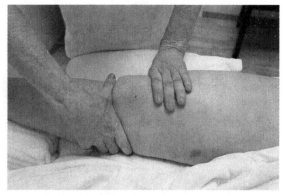

a. Wringing the kneecap

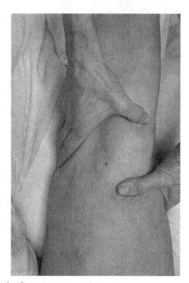

b. Slicing the kneecap

Figure 2.20. Wringing and slicing around the kneecap really helps relieve tension in the knees. Pregnancy hormones make the mom's joints more mobile. That extra mobility, plus weight gain, often gives women knee problems during pregnancy.

8. **Alternate thumb kneading to the upper leg**: Use this stroke on the head of the femur, on the quadriceps, and around the kneecap.

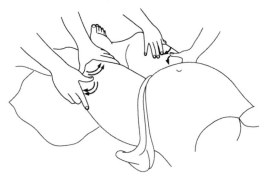

Figure 2.21. Alternate thumb kneading to the quadriceps.

When I knead the head of the femur, I turn my body so I am facing the side of the leg. This way I can work with power behind the stroke. Do alternate thumb kneading all around the head of the femur. The stroke is very good for working out sore spots, kneading them into submission. After massaging all around the side of the hip, start down the leg along the iliotibial band.

When you massage down the iliotibial band, step back and stride out so your back leg is way behind you. When you lean into your front leg (like you are starting out in a sprint position), you are able to get a lot of power behind your thumbs.

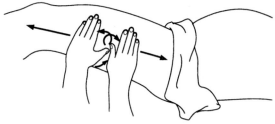

Figure 2.22. Alternate thumb kneading to the iliotibial band. Massage from the hip to the outside of the knee.

Transition: Alternate thumb kneading moves from the upper leg and hip, thigh, and knee to the lower leg, where it becomes even more appreciated, even in the first trimester. This is where the symptoms of the changes in vascular activity are most strongly felt first.

9. **Alternate thumb kneading to the lower leg**: The tiny alternate thumb-kneading strokes are perfectly designed for the tibialis anterior muscle. This is the long sinewy muscle running down the front of the lower leg alongside the ridge of the tibia (shin bone) into the foot. The muscle is often associated with shin splints. The alternate thumb kneading of this muscle is small and very focused. Both thumbs stay on the outside of the ridge, and I stay on the tips of my thumbs. The stroke gives immediate relief to lower-leg congestion and greater flexibility in the ankle.

10. **Wringing to the lower leg**: Be sure to include the gastrocnemius (calf muscle), the ankle, and the foot. I use a grip that goes around the corners of the malleoli (ankles bones) and then wring across the foot.

11. **Effleurage**: Finish with effleurage to the full leg or just the lower leg, moving to the foot effleurage. Be sure to lean firmly onto the sole of the foot when you begin the final effleurages.

FEET AND ANKLES (SUPINE)

I spend extra time at the feet; although they are rarely a problem in the first trimester, they are a source of heavy-duty relaxation. Although these directions are described as though the mom is lying supine, you can massage her feet when she is in any position. The strokes are highly adaptable.

1. **Mini-effleurage**: Place your hands in a prayer position sandwiching the foot with one hand across the sole of the foot and the other hand across the top. Move this prayerful sandwich up and down the foot with the emphasis on pushing into the bottom of the foot with the heel of your hand. This is done at least three times (but because it is usually a huge favorite, it could be done 100 times).

2. **Kneading to the malleoli**: Use the heels of your hands to knead the malleoli (ankle bones) of each foot. Cup the foot in both hands and knead the malleoli with your thumbs, one thumb on the outer malleolus and the other thumb on the inner malleolus. You can also do this in an alternating movement of the thumbs.

3. **Alternate thumb kneading to the top and sole of the foot**: Cupping the foot, thumb knead the top and sole of the foot. On the sole, alternate thumb kneading will help erase the aches and pains of the day or, in pregnancy, of the hour! Massage slowly and firmly if the mom is ticklish.

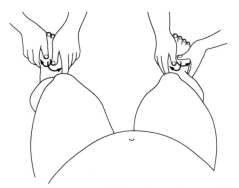

Figure 2.24. Alternate thumb kneading to the top of the foot.

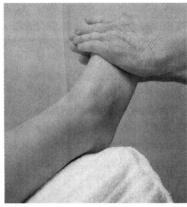

Figure 2.23. A prayer sandwich.

4. **Thumb wringing to the top and sole of the foot**: Push your thumbs toward each other across the foot first on the top and then on the sole. The thumbs should cross paths right beside each other as they push out to the edges of the foot on opposite sides and then pull back across. This back and forth movement, which runs against the grain of the muscles, feels great from the first trimester to the last.

To wring across the sole of the foot, you may want to drop down to your knees to kneel or squat at the mom's feet. After thumb wringing, try some alternating digital compression to the area, pressing slowly with your thumbs like a kneading cat all over the bottom of the foot.

5. **Toe corkscrewing**: Wring the toes one by one with a corkscrewing technique toward the nearest side of the foot, so two toes will be wrung in one direction and two toes in the opposite direction, with the middle toe able to go either way or both directions.

   Do this tiny outward wringing motion as slowly as you can, three times for each toe. To get the right balance, be sure to change hands and go one direction with one hand toward the outside of the foot, then change hands and do the same thing on the other side. After the wringing is done, another effleurage can be used to connect to the next strokes in the progression of increasing pressure and focus.

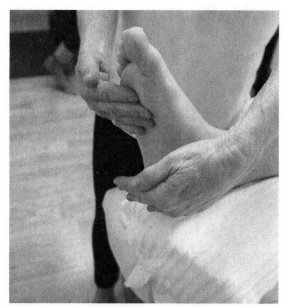

Figure 2.26. For percussive rolling on the bottom of the foot, you can use tightly rolled fists or open, flat hands.

7. **Light reflex stroking**: Finish off with light reflex stroking to the entire leg.

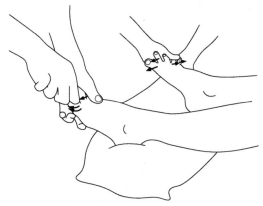

Figure 2.25. Wring each toe to the nearest edge of the foot. The middle toe can go either or both ways.

6. **Percussive rolling to the sole of the foot**: Stand at the side of the table facing away from the mom, looking down at her feet. With your hands in tight fists, apply a pounding stroke to the sole of the foot with a rolling, Ferris wheel motion. See page 24 for details on pounding tapotement.

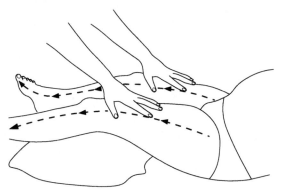

Figure 2.27. Finish with light reflex stroking to the legs, from feet to hips.

ARMS (SUPINE)

1. **Effleurage**: Stroke three times up the arm with both hands beside each other, or use one hand and then the other. Whichever method you use, pressure goes up the arm from hand to shoulder, with no pressure on the way down.

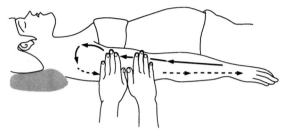

a. Two hands effleurage as one unit.

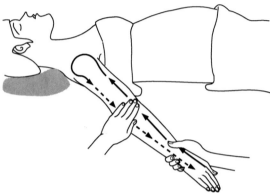

b. Hold the wrist with one hand. Effleurage up the outside of the arm, loop around the shoulder, and return to the hand without pressure.

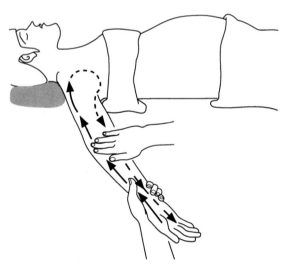

c. Hold the wrist with one hand. Effleurage up the inside of the arm to the armpit and return to the hand without pressure.

Figure 2.28. Arm effleurage can be done with two hands together or one hand at a time.

2. **Single-handed palmar kneading to the deltoids:** Hold the arm by the wrist and knead the deltoid muscle at the top of the shoulder with the other hand.

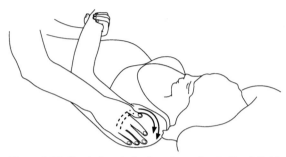

Figure 2.29. Single-handed palmar kneading to the deltoid muscle.

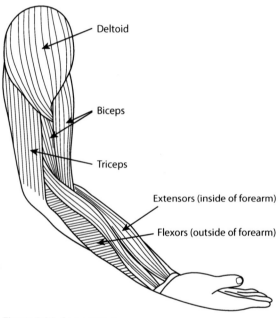

Figure 2.30. Arm anatomy.

3. **Reinforced palmar kneading to the pectorals:** With one palm on top of the other, knead the shoulder from the front pushing toward the back, stretching out the pectorals (chest muscles). Two other options for palmar kneading to the pectorals are shown in Figures 2.31 and 2.32.

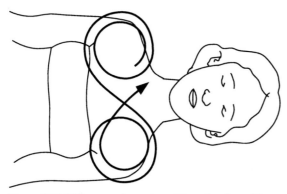

Figure 2.31. With one palm on top of the other, knead the pectorals in a figure eight with pressure pushing from the front to the back.

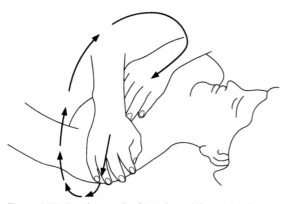

Figure 2.32. Another method is to knead the pectorals away from you using overhanded palmar kneading.

4. **Single-handed thumb kneading to the triceps:** Hold the wrist with your inner hand and knead the triceps with the thumb of your other hand.

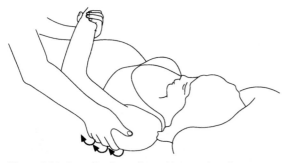

Figure 2.33. As well as kneading with your thumbs, you can use a small C-shape of your hand to scoop up and release the triceps.

5. **Alternate thumb kneading to the biceps:** Let the forearm rest up against your body, or it can be lying down straight. Knead the biceps with your thumbs.

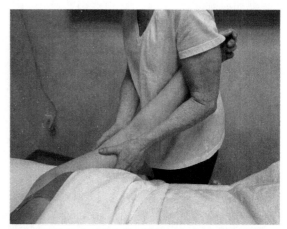

Figure 2.34. You can rest the forearm against your body to knead the biceps.

6. **Palmar kneading to the elbow bump:** With your inside hand, hold the wrist and bend the arm. Cup the olecranon (elbow bump) with your other hand and knead it with a circular motion.

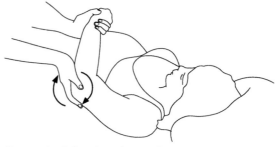

Figure 2.35. Palmar kneading to elbow.

7. **Alternate thumb kneading to the inner elbow:** This is the delicious part of the arm massage for all trimesters and postpartum. Spend lots of time at the inner elbow with slow alternate thumb kneading and possibly some thumb wringing.
8. **Effleurage to the forearm.**
9. **Alternate thumb kneading to the forearm:** Lean the forearm against your tummy

and knead the inner-arm flexors with your thumbs. Then knead the forearm extensors on the back of the forearm, working slowly and firmly toward the hand.

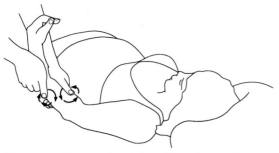

Figure 2.36. Alternate thumb kneading to forearm flexors.

10. **Single-handed thumb kneading to the forearm**: Hold the wrist with one hand and knead the forearm with the other. Alternate your hands so each massages both outer and inner arm.

11. **Alternate thumb kneading to the back of the hand**: The hand is important to massage as the mom's rings will start to feel tight at three months. Bend the arm at the elbow and wrist and support the arm on the table. Start with alternate thumb kneading to the top (back) of the hand.

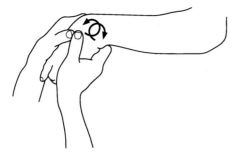

Figure 2.37. Alternate thumb kneading to the back of the hand. Start at the wrist for some focused attention.

12. **Corkscrew the fingers**: With the fingers pointing toward you, corkscrew each finger individually, with emphasis on each joint. Make it a continuous motion from the base to the tip of each finger using the same system you used

for the toes. Wring the thumb toward the outside of the hand. (It just doesn't feel right to do it the other way—try it and see!) Each finger will have a natural feel for which way to wring it, but my design is to do each of the outside fingers to their respective sides and the middle finger can go either (or both) ways.

13. **Alternate thumb kneading to the palm**: Now do some alternate thumb kneading to the palm. Hold the hand up with the arm bent and forearm leaning on the table. Bend the wrist back so the fingers are pointing up. Knead the entire palmar surface of the hand, focusing on the base of each finger and the heel of the hand and thumb. This is often the most relaxing part of the arm massage.

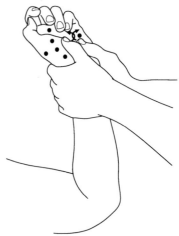

Figure 2.38. Alternate thumb kneading to the palm of the hand. You can also do some digital compression.

14. **Effleurage the arm**: Stroke the entire arm up and down three times.

15. **Light reflex stroking**: Finish with light reflex stroking. Alternate your hands running lightly down the arm without pressure from shoulder to fingertips. The movement is continuous, with one hand starting the stroke at the shoulder just as the other finishes at the fingertips. Do each arm at least three times. From the arm massage, you can move to the front of the body.

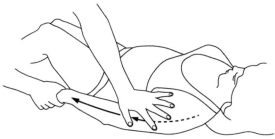

Figure 2.39. Light reflex stroking to the arm.

ABDOMEN

1. **Effleurage**: There are two different styles and starting positions. Whichever style you choose, effleurage the trunk of the body from chest to stomach three times. In the first trimester, there will not be a big tummy to accommodate in this stroke, but you may have some breast draping to hop over with the full-frontal effleurage.

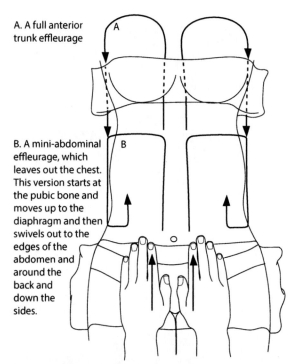

A. A full anterior trunk effleurage

B. A mini-abdominal effleurage, which leaves out the chest. This version starts at the pubic bone and moves up to the diaphragm and then swivels out to the edges of the abdomen and around the back and down the sides.

Figure 2.40. Anterior trunk effleurage.

- **From lower abdomen up**: Start this stroke standing at the side of the table, facing the mom's head. Put one foot ahead of the other: the outside leg is ahead in a stride position. Place your hands gently, with the fingers pointing up toward the mom's head, on the lower part of the abdomen and head up the center of the tummy to the sternum, out the clavicle (collarbone), around the deltoid muscle at the top of the arms, and then back down the sides to the starting point. As you come back down to the starting position, you can let your hands glide around the back of the mom with a bit of a lifting action.
- **From sternum down**: Stand at the mom's head and place both hands on the sternum, facing the toes. Head down the abdomen, circle around, and pull up the sides to loop around the shoulders to the start. Again, you can let your backstroke move around to the back of the mom and ease up any back tension on your return.

2. **Wringing across the abdomen**: Pull and push your hands across the abdomen, gently wringing the skin of the pregnant tummy between the pubic bone and the diaphragm. Wedge your hands closely together so some real wringing can happen. I don't use as much pressure in my abdominal wringing as I do on the legs, but it is still a worthwhile stroke to include in the abdominal massage.

3. **Overhanded palmar kneading to the digestive tract**: Using the entire palmar surface of your hands, do large circles following the digestive tract up the right side and across at the ribs and down the left side. Glide without pressure across the lower aspect at the bladder. Follow the first hand with the second, hopping over each other in a continuous motion. The right hand stays on the whole time doing continuous circles while the left hand hops over. You can do this three to thirty times!

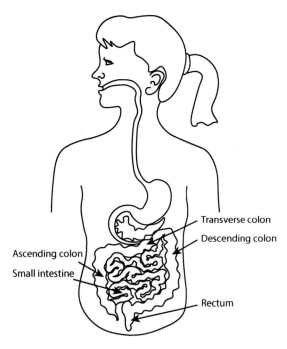

Transverse colon

Descending colon

Ascending colon

Small intestine

Rectum

Figure 2.41. Follow the direction of the digestive tract to encourage a sluggish system to get moving.

4. **Reinforced fingertip kneading to the digestive tract**: Use reinforced fingertip kneading along the path of the digestive tract. Pause in each of the four corners for at least a minute. Take it slowly, and do the whole square at least three times. You can start at the descending colon and work backward, or start at the ascending colon and work forward. Either way works.

5. **Wringing across the abdomen**: Wring across the abdomen again to "erase" the focused attention of the fingertip kneading.

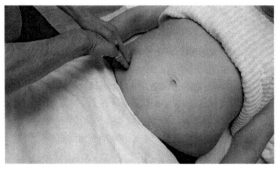

a.

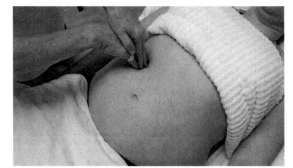

b.

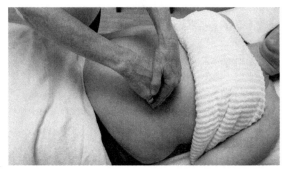

c.

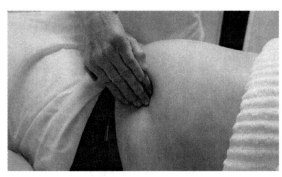

d.

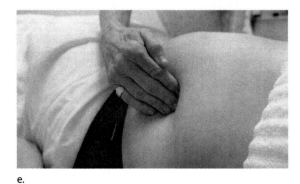

e.

Figure 2.42. Fingertip kneading to the digestive tract. Be sure to be on the tips of your fingers for the best benefits.

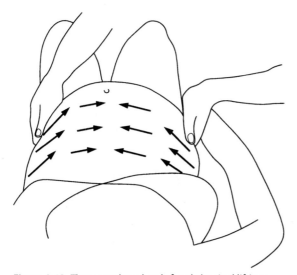

Figure 2.43. There are three levels for abdominal lifting: low back, waistline, and ribs.

6. **Abdominal lifting**: Do abdominal lifting at three levels: around the diaphragm, around the waistline, and around the low back. If you are working on the bed or floor, be sure to use the one-knee-up and one-knee-down posture (shiatsu position). Make sure your knee down is the one next to the patient. When working with the person on a table, lean against the table to stabilize your back. Reach around to the back with a hand on either side of her body. Meet your fingertips at the spine and then slowly lift, pulling up and out. This stroke gives a nice stretch to her back. You can make the effect more therapeutic by making it very, very slow, and then the effort to get underneath is rewarded by the stroke being longer lasting and extra penetrating in its effect.

7. **Overhanded palmar kneading around the digestive tract**: Repeat this three times.

8. **Effleurage**: Do three effleurage strokes to the abdomen.

9. **Light reflex stroking**: Use your fingertips with no pressure, just contact.

Transition: If I'm moving from the abdomen directly to a breast massage, I add in a full-frontal effleurage to put the whole trunk of the person back into play. I end up at the

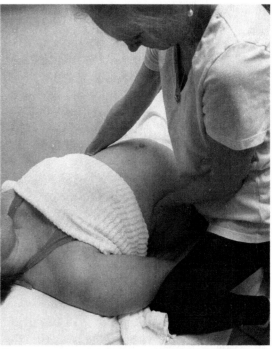

Figure 2.44. Place a knee up on the bed or table to protect your back as you reach under the mom.

shoulders for reinforced palmar kneading to the shoulders in the shape of a large figure eight. I then add in some reinforced fingertip kneading to the lower aspect of the collarbone where the breasts are starting to grow.

BREASTS

Breast changes in the first trimester can be uncomfortable, and this massage of three strokes helps reduce discomfort and raise awareness of the changing breasts. See chapter 6 for a thorough discussion of breast massage pre- and postpartum.

1. **Effleurage**: Two versions of the effleurage are described below; whichever you choose, do it three times to start the breast massage. I like to do both versions, changing my position in between.

   - **From shoulders down**: Stand at the head of the mom and place both hands on the upper chest at the shoulders, palms down, and head toward the middle of the sternum, then push down the center lane between the breasts and circle around to the outside at the rib cage. Swivel your hands out to the mom's sides, sliding your fingers underneath her. Pull back toward yourself with firm pressure, keeping your fingers together underneath her and your palms up her sides until you reach the armpits. Your hands can then loop around the sides of the breasts to the starting point. A relaxing alternative is to move from the armpits to the outside of the shoulder and then loop around the back of the deltoid muscle at the upper arm where it connects to the trunk of the body. Continue up the back of the neck to end the stroke. Lift your hands and put them back to the starting position at the front of the shoulder.

- **From diaphragm up**: Face-to-face with the mom, start at the bottom, right at the level of the diaphragm. Move up the center with two hands fitting between the breasts beside each other. Go to the top and then head out to the shoulders and loop generously toward the back around the shoulders and come down the sides, without pulling on the breasts, in a downward motion.

2. **Scooping**: With a C-shaped cup shape to the hands, scoop the breast in an upward direction toward the middle, letting go before you hit the nipple. Use an alternating motion,

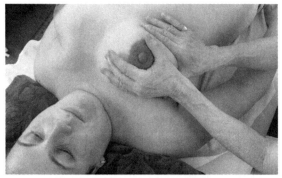

a. With alternating hands in an open C-shape, scoop the breast without making contact with the nipple. Scoop from the armpit area and the side of the mother.

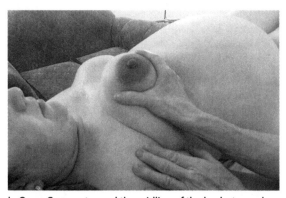

b. Open C scoop toward the midline of the body, toward the center of the breastbone.

Figure 2.46. The trick with the scooping stroke is to let the breast slip through and not to touch, grip, or make any other contact with the nipple. Just concentrate on the breast itself. You want to focus on massaging the ducts and lymph nodes and the general circulation of the breast.

scooping with each hand, with one hand letting go just as the other hand starts. It is a gentle tossing of the breast from one hand to the other. Do this at least ten times to each breast.

3. **Reinforced fingertip kneading**: Do reinforced fingertip kneading to the attachments of the pectoral muscles where they insert into the sternum and the arm and below the collarbone. Move in a figure-eight pattern around the breasts. You may need to hold the breast out of the way with one hand, which will make the other hand do single-handed fingertip

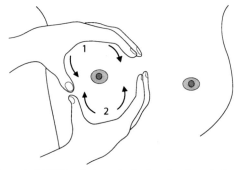

Figure 2.45. With a C-shape to the hands, alternate hands to scoop up into the center of the breast, taking care not to touch the nipple.

kneading. As always, pressure of the individual strokes is upward. These strokes can be soothing to the breasts, which may be hypersensitive during this first trimester.

4. **Scooping**: Repeat the scooping three times minimum to each breast.

5. **Effleurage**: Repeat the effleurage strokes three times in either direction. Cover the whole trunk, from chest to abdomen.

The breast massage can be combined with the abdominal massage, before the abdominal massage, after the abdominal massage, or before and after! After finishing, I like to place a hot water bottle on the mom's tummy and tuck her in with blankets or sheets before beginning the face and scalp routine as the finishing touch to the full-body massage.

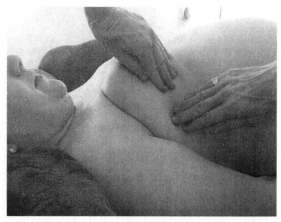

Figure 2.49. On the outer side of the breasts, you may need to use single-handed fingertip kneading so the other hand can hold the breast away from the sag down.

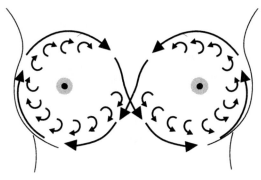

Figure 2.47. Path of reinforced fingertip and single-handed fingertip kneading around the breasts. Always apply pressure in an upward direction—never downward.

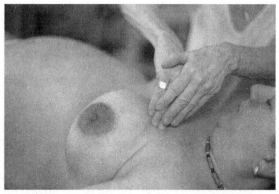

Figure 2.48. Stack your fingertips on top of each other so that one hand is on top of the other. Keep the fingers straight, not bent. Now pivot your wrist. The arch of the hand is bent at the base of the fingers so they stay straight and the pivoting action originates at the wrist.

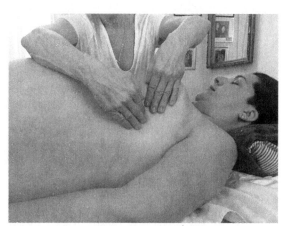

Figure 2.50. As you go around the breast on the far side (the breast furthest away from you) make sure your reinforced fingertip kneading is done in an upward direction, massaging where the breast attaches to the body. One hand should hold the breast up out of the way while the other hand does the fingertip kneading along that side. At about the level of the armpit, the breast can be let go so you can stack your fingers up again and continue around the top to the changeover in the center on the sternum.

FACE AND SCALP

The face and scalp massage can alleviate headaches and will help your mom relax or sleep better. Patient positioning for this massage is supine, lying face up on any surface, including the couch, bed, or floor.

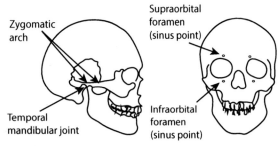

Figure 2.51. Face anatomy.

1. **Head flexion**: Standing at the head of the table (if the mom is lying on a table) lift the head three times very slowly, chin to chest. Coach the mom to relax the weight of her head in your hands. (Figure 2.52a)

2. **Scalp kneading**: Slowly and firmly use your fingertips to knead the scalp. You should be able to see the mom's forehead wrinkling as you do this. Keep moving to a new location and get a new grip, but do not rub back and forth or you will wear out your welcome! Hook onto the scalp and move it with no frictioning back and forth. (Figure 2.52b)

   Slowly turn the head to one side with a hand under one ear. Use your free hand to slowly and deliberately knead the scalp at the back of the head on the occipital ridge. Slowly turn the head to the other side, again holding a hand under the ear, and use the other fingertips to firmly and slowly knead. (Figure 2.52c)

   Keep asking the mom on the receiving end about pressure (i.e., "Can I press firmer?" "Should I lighten up?"). These questions will get you further than simply asking how it is going, which will result in answers such as "Fine," or "Great," but will not give you the information you need about increasing or decreasing pressure. Ask the right questions

to get the right answers, as this massage can relieve a pregnancy headache in a minute of just the right pressure.

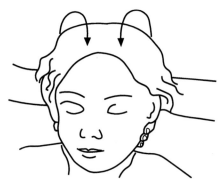

a. Lift the head three times. Coach the mom to let her head drop into your hands, not help!

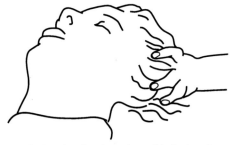

b. Rotate the head and make a claw with the hands so you can massage the scalp with your fingertips. Be firm and check in frequently.

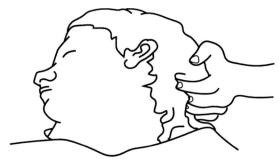

c. Fingertip knead to the base of the skull with an upward traction in each stroke at the attachments. This will help lessen tension in the mom's neck.

Figure 2.52. Scalp massage.

3. **Facial contour stroking**: Sitting at the head of the mom, or facing her, wipe any hair from the scalp massage off your hands in a visible

way so the mom knows you are not tracking hair all over her face. Be sure to keep your nails really short because this stroke uses the tips of the fingers to contour the face.

- **Lower contour stroking**: Line up your fingertips alongside each other so they will act as one unit. Start in the middle of the face with a hand on each side of the centerline. From this start, slowly stretch the contours of the face from the center out to the ears and temples. Do each contour at least three times. Begin at the lower and then upper ridge of the chinline. Pull out toward the temples in an upward direction. Then start at the midline right below the lips. Then stroke above the lips, again starting in the middle of the face and moving out along the contour of the face to the ear and temples (along the zygomatic arch).

    Moving up the face, start at the outer flare of the nostrils and again firmly glide your fingertips along that ridge out to the temples. Now start at the bridge of the nose and stroke along the lower orbit of the eye. The last stroke starts right between the eyes and again goes along the lower border of the eye. You may be able to feel the sinus point in the midline of the edge of the eye as you pull by it. (Figure 2.53a)

- **Upper contour stroking**: The contours of the upper face are stroked with the thumbs, starting in the center between the eyes on the eyebrows. Slowly, using steady pressure, stroke along the eyebrows. With each stroke, move a little higher toward the hairline, dividing the forehead into about four or five levels of contour stroking with the thumbs. Move slowly and deliberately. Keep your direction always heading outward toward the temples and collect each stroke in that area with some fingertip kneading. Do the entire forehead sequence three times. (Figure 2.53b)

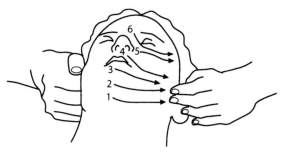

a. Lower contour stroking

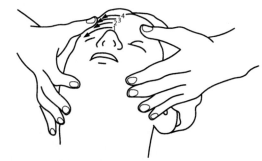

b. Upper contour stroking

Figure 2.53. Face stroking.

4. **Kneading to the jaw**: Ask the mom to relax her jaw so you can knead around the temporal mandibular joint and down the jaw toward the chin with your fingertips.

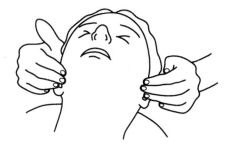

Figure 2.54. Knead at the temporal mandibular joint in front of the lower earlobes.

5. **Fingertip kneading to the temples**: Press the tips of your three middle fingers together on the temples, right on the hairline where the skin and scalp meet. Along this line of tissue change, the sensitivity is acute, so you get a good relaxation response. Keep your fingers

straight and allow your wrists to pivot so you get greater precision by being right on the tips of the fingers. From here it is easy to move along to the ear massage.

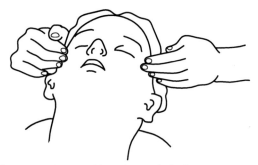

Figure 2.55. Temporal kneading with the fingertips.

6. **Fingertip kneading to the ears:** Work both sides at the same time with fingertip kneading at the attachment of the ears to the sides of the head. Massage with the tips of your fingers in the crease with firm pressure. Go three times around the ear in each direction, for six times total. Although everyone tends to bend their fingers in this stroke, try to keep your fingers straight so they contact less of the skin surface. For maximum benefit, be on the tips of straight fingers.

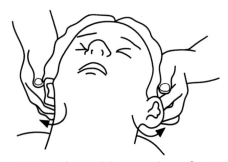

Figure 2.56. Knead around the ears with your fingertips.

Again check in about pressure. Sometimes if the person is or was a smoker or is a big smiler, then this massage will elicit a coughing response, which is a great compliment to the therapist. This focused massage will get those smiling muscles loosened up in the temporal mandibular joint as you come around the

front of the ear. Switch directions as you travel around the ear to balance the sensation; go in one direction and then reverse and do the fingertip kneading in the other direction.

7. **Passive ear rotations:** Grasp an ear in each hand. Give a slight traction by pulling outward, rotate the ears with steady pulling in one direction three times, and then reverse and go in the other direction (Figure 2.57). You can change this for variety by alternating the movements back and forth between the ears and then ending with fingertip kneading around the ear attachments to the side of the head.

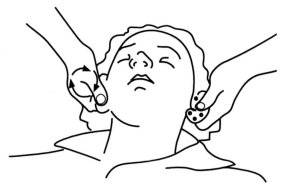

Figure 2.57. Ear rotations and pressure points.

8. **Roll-through fingertip kneading to the edge of the ear:** Start anywhere along the outer edge of the ear flap and roll the edge between your thumb against the rest of your fingers. It is a bit like the hand signal for money in which you roll your thumb against your other fingers. Once you get the hang of it, the mom will love it. This stroke is one my patients tell each other about—a favorite.

The best spot to do this is the lobe of the ear. Because pregnant women are notoriously hypersensitive, these outer reaches of the body are like whiskers for sensing touch! The pregnant mom will purr for you to keep massaging her ears in this spot.

This stroke is not only good for headaches, but also for C-sections; while the medical crew is organizing, I work away on the mom's head and ears, which are out of sight so it doesn't look obvious that I am massaging my patient. It looks like a tender touch, but it packs a really big impact on the body. Ears are well built for focused attention from tiny massage strokes.

9. **Digital compression to the outer ear**: Use your pointer finger and thumb to squeeze or pinch around the outer perimeter of the ear. This will give the ear a tingly feeling. Press slowly and firmly and ask the mom how it feels. Slower is better as it allows her time to digest the stroke and gives the stroke more time to make an impression. Work around the entire edge of the ear three times. This stroke is used in Chinese ear acupressure.

10. **Ear roll-through**: Repeat the ear roll-through three times.

11. **Shampoo fingertip kneading**: This is the wake-up call for the person on the receiving end to come back to life, but a warning: this stroke will give a brand-new, electrifying hairdo! Hold the head with one hand and with great speed, rub back and forth in a dryland shampoo massage. It is a vigorous movement that makes fur fly with a polishing type of stroke back and forth across the scalp: superficial, yet stimulating at the same time.

This has to be done lightly enough to not cause problems by irritating the hair follicles. Ask the mom how she feels and she will tell you that she loves it. Ask about pressure: "Should I go firmer or lighter?" Be sure to turn the head to one side slowly, although your other shampooing hand is moving quickly. After doing the back of the head by turning the face from side to side (remembering to keep the hand under the head for stability), position the person's head face-up again and start to slow the stroke down using a hand on either side of the head and scalp. Stop when you have covered the whole scalp. (Figure 2.58)

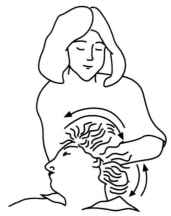

Figure 2.58. Shampoo massage.

12. **Fingertip kneading to the scalp**: Begin to gear down to a slow, focused fingertip kneading. With your hands in a claw-like position, work one area and then move to a new spot, working along the whole scalp. Ask again about pressure: "Should I go firmer or lighter?"

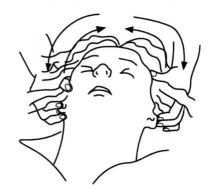

Figure 2.59. Fingertip kneading to scalp.

13. **Light stroking**: With the tips of the fingers, stroke the face from the center to the outside edge. Do this at least three times. Then try the same direction of stroke using the back of the fingers, making the stroke lighter and lighter. This is an excellent headache remedy. It has a mesmerizing effect that is also good for labor and delivery between contractions while someone else is massaging the arms and legs. This stroking for the face is a great way to keep someone calm and collected during an existentially stressful time. (Figure 2.60)

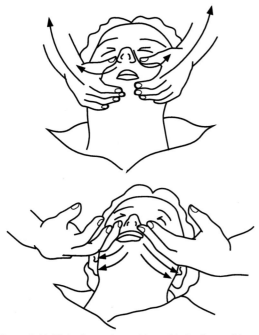

Figure 2.60. Light fingertip stroking with the front of the fingers and then the back of the fingers.

14. **Fingertip butterfly massage:** Using the fingertips only, tap along the cheeks with straight fingertips, like stiff-fingered piano playing. This is a favorite stroke I learned from my friend Catherine. It has become the closing benediction of my face-and-scalp routine that is usually at the end of my full-body massages. Ask the massaged person to take at least twenty-seven deep breaths and just drift.

15. **Facial cupping:** Another nice finish is to rub your hands together quickly to warm them and then cup the face firmly. Do this three times as the mom takes three deep breaths.

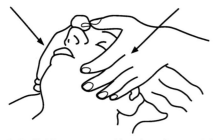

Figure 2.61. Hold your warmed hands to the mom's face as she breathes deeply.

Second Trimester Massage

During the second trimester, pregnant women are beginning to bloom into full pregnancy mode. The pregnancy "bump" is more apparent and, as the baby grows, so do the pressures on the mom's body to accommodate it. However, the common symptoms of the second trimester are massageable and manageable. They range from headaches to back pain and sometimes sciatica. I find that my patients are usually coming for professional help because the amateur massages they are getting at home need a boost.

"My second trimester massages are the best way to soothe the body, take time for me, and connect with baby! Plus I'm learning the tools to help prevent the symptoms of heartburn and sciatica that I had endured with my first pregnancy." —Nadine

Timing

Aim for one professional massage per week, plus daily massages from friends and family.

Patient positioning

Somewhere in the second trimester, the mom will want to transition to a side-lying position for massage. The massage directions below are for side-lying massage. Turn to pages 28–29 for specific directions for pillow positioning.

Massage for the second trimester

BACK (SIDE-LYING)

1. **Effleurage:** Each hand is on either side of the spine if the person can lie so that both sides of her back are exposed, but I can't always get to the downside closest to the massage surface equally as well. Sometimes I can only do the upper side of the person's back and then I turn the person over and repeat so I can balance the two sides. It is like doing two back massages put together into one!

There are two kinds of effleurage for a side-lying back massage:

- **From the top of the back toward the sacrum**: Starting at the shoulders, lean down the back, with one hand on either side of the spine from the top of the shoulders to the lowest part of the back that I can reach. I find that effleuraging down the back gives me more stretching power for the aches and pains of my patients' low back. Really emphasize the downward pressure on the lumbar and sacral areas and take that part as slowly as possible before you return up the sides to your starting point on top of the trapezius at the head, neck, and shoulders.

- **From the sacrum upward to the neck and shoulders**: Starting at the sacrum, follow the ropy erector spinae muscles up the spine to the base of the skull at the occipital-ridge attachments. Then turn out toward the shoulders and arms, massaging with your palmar surface down the sides to start again at the sacrum. Working these muscles from one end to the other is important. Effleurage with the entire palmar aspect of your hands, including the fingers to the tips.

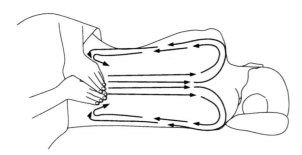

Figure 2.62. Effleurage from the sacrum up the spine.

Whichever direction you massage, put both hands on the back and lean your body weight onto them. You can step alongside the table as you move to keep your body weight on the hands. To get the right angle, wedge one or both elbows into your body and use that levering pressure to slowly press and glide up or down her back, with one hand on either side of her spine.

The mom probably needs about one hundred of these long, firm effleurage strokes! Be sure to check in with her about how firm to go and how many she needs before you move along to the next stroke. Do at least three before moving on. I usually move from effleurage to a couple of other broad-handed strokes, collecting information about the mom's condition and deciding where to concentrate my attention.

2. **Wringing**: You can do this wringing facing the mom's back or you can do it from the mom's front reaching over her. Most commonly I do this stroke from the back of the patient, but in the hospital, I will sometimes apply it from the front if we have lots of people working together or some restriction in access to her back. (Figure 2.63)

Step back from the massage table to get the right posture to do this wringing stroke from the back. Take a stride position like you are starting a race with one leg out in front of the other, the front knee bent. Lean forward to put pressure onto your hands. The palms are the massaging part of the hand, with a cupping curve that conforms to the shape of the mom's back as you wring up and down. Make sure that your hands brush by each other with each wringing movement. If they are not touching each other, the wringing action will not be as effective in breaking the surface tension of the skin.

So don't be generous and cover the whole back with divorced-hands wringing. Marry those two hands together and push and pull the tension out of the back from the shoulders and upper back to the achy low back. As you wring the back in side-lying, you have to really bend your wrists to get down to the surface the mom is lying on. This can be pretty awkward, so you may find it easier to wring the top side of the back first (from spine to top) and then wring the other side after the mom flips over. (Figure 2.64)

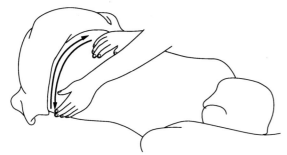

Figure 2.63. Bilateral wringing.

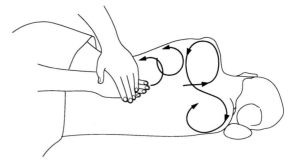

Figure 2.65. Reinforced palmar kneading.

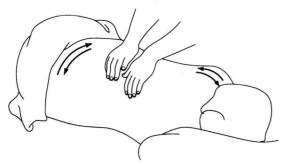

Figure 2.64. Unilateral wringing to back and shoulders.

Working across the direction of the muscle fibers seems to provide an extra-pleasant sensation. At the same time, it is a highly effective therapeutic stroke, especially for the shoulders when you put two hands to work wringing one shoulder and then the other in turn.

3. **Reinforced palmar kneading**: This stroke uses your whole body weight in a rocking action. Get into a stride position alongside the table facing toward the head of the table. Stack your hands one on top of the other. Switch hands from top to bottom to see which is more comfortable or gives you the greatest power.

   Start at either the lower or upper back, it doesn't matter, but make the circular strokes small enough that it takes five or six circles to travel up or down one side. Be careful not to knead on the spine itself and to keep the direction of pressure up and out, away from the spine.

   When you move to the other side of the spine with this stroke, do a figure-eight pattern at the shoulders or the low back,

wherever you need to switch directions. So if I've been massaging from low back to shoulders, at the top of the back I do a figure eight with my hands, traveling from the side I've been massaging to the opposite side, always making the direction of pressure up and away from the spine. Once I knead down the other side, at the low back I do another figure eight before I start up the other side again.

Be sure to use the stride position to protect your back and get enough pressure for your strokes.

Repeat this entire cycle of kneading three or four times, being sure to cover the shoulders and checking in about the pressure. Even if the mom can turn from side to side, I still include the lower aspect of the back (the side closest to the table). Then when the person turns over and I repeat the massage, both sides will be balanced, receiving a massage from the top side and bottom side.

Now you can use the tiny drill strokes of frictioning, thumb stroking, alternate thumb kneading, and reinforced fingertip kneading anywhere on the back that has tight spots.

4. **Thumb stroking**: Apply this long, continuous stroke to the entire length of the spine in the natural groove between the erector spinae muscles and the spine. Just fit your thumb into this groove and slide it along. Use one thumb at a time, moving slowly and deeply.

   Work from as high up on the neck as possible down to where the groove ends as the erector spinae muscles attach to the sacrum. You may need to adapt the angle of your arm and hand to keep the stroke moving steadily up or down the mom's back. This stroke is also good if the mom can lie prone. With either patient positioning, this stroke has great releasing potential. I usually do this stroke from three to five times once I have the area loosened up by the other introductory strokes.

5. **Alternate thumb kneading**: Now it's time to let loose on those shoulder and back muscles! The first place I focus my attention is on the low back, where the second-trimester weight gain can cause problems. But I also use kneading along the erector spinae muscles, all over the shoulder area, and on the hips.

   Alternate thumb kneading is the main course of massage strokes. The stroke is all thumbs, but the hands and fingers provide tripod support for the thumbs as they work away on the muscles. Move your thumbs in small, focused, overlapping circles with pressure up and out in opposing mirrors.

   Ask the mom where her sore spots are as this stroke is the best way to unwind some big problems. These strokes are like tiny drills that pave the way to the deeper strokes of reinforced fingertip kneading and frictioning.

6. **Reinforced fingertip kneading**: With one set of fingers on top of the other, keeping the fingers straight with the wrists pivoting on the fingertips, work in circular movements up the same path as the alternate thumb kneading in an outward direction of pressure away from the spine. Pay special attention to the low back, the rhomboids, and the trapezius muscles. By this time, you will know where the mom's favorite spots are, and you can work them out with this stroke. Check in with the mom to see if she finds this stroke or the thumbs more effective.

7. **Intermittent digital thumb compression**: This is another favorite stroke for working the back. Standing in a stride position, use straight thumbs to press with one thumb and then the other, right then left, working away like a kneading cat all along the length of the erector spinae muscles.

   This is a great way to break up any remaining tension and spasticity in the back muscles. It is also my best stroke for working the hips in a side-lying position. I can spend a long time working away at the back with this "poke-and-press" routine.

8. **Frictioning for adhesions**: Use this vigorous back and forth movement to drill on any adhesions to break them down and make the muscle tissue more elastic and expandable.

9. **Counterpressure for trigger points**: A trigger point is a hypersensitive area on the body that can sometimes be felt as a lumpy or fibrous spot. Trigger points give a great opportunity to practice the breathing exercises and verbal commands for counterpressure on the sacrum that you will want to use during labor and delivery.

   If you locate a trigger point along the back, put your thumb into the spot with steady pressure. Ask the mom to breathe into the sensation until it disappears or feels like you are lightening up on the pressure. After about four or five deep breaths, check in and ask if the sensation is starting to subside. Usually it is, but if it isn't, then I know I'm not in the right place or my angle isn't accurate. If this happens, adjust your angle or shift slightly in the spot with feedback from the mom.

   "Let me know when I get that spot right on" is my frequent request to my pregnant patient. The Sutherland approach is using the F-word: feedback, feedback, feedback! for the best touch.

   When you have worked on three or four trigger points along the back or in the shoulders, then you are ready to ask the mom to flip over to the other side for the same massage sequence. Before turning, erase the trigger-point muscle memory by finishing with your progression of strokes in reverse (trigger points » wringing » effleurage) so no thumbprints remain in the mom's muscle memory.

Remember to balance the back with equal time on each side. Fifteen minutes per side is perfect. I will almost always do both sides in each side-lying position, but some people cannot be on one side and then the other; they are only comfortable on one side. With these folks, I do the massage in its entirety on the one side, and work underneath them as well as I can by levering my fingertips on the bed to knead the side of the body that is lying against the table or bed.

10. Effleurage and light reflex stroking to finish.

Transition: After the back, you have a choice about where you can go: to the arms or legs.

HIPS AND LEGS (SIDE-LYING)

The side-lying hip massage is one of the best ways to really get into the hip area and loosen it up. The side-lying position exposes more attachments and gives greater accessibility to the entire hip area. Even if the mom is comfortable on her back, I will often get her to lie on her side for greater effectiveness.

WHEN YOUR SIDE-LYING PATIENT CAN'T LIE ON THE OTHER SIDE

If the mom I'm massaging in side-lying isn't able to flip over to her other side, I can still do both legs. Once I finish the leg on top, I ask the mom to straighten the lower leg if it is bent in full-crooked position. When the bottom leg is straight, I can massage it with the same sequence of strokes, working the hip by sliding my hands underneath and levering my fingertips up into the hip joint. That lower leg need not be left out! Even if you cannot achieve a perfect balance, you can manage an effective massage for the lower leg.

1. **Effleurage from toes to hip**: Effleurage up the leg from the toes to the hip with pressure, turn your hands at the head of the femur, and then glide back down without pressure, just good contact. Doing effleurage is quite different on

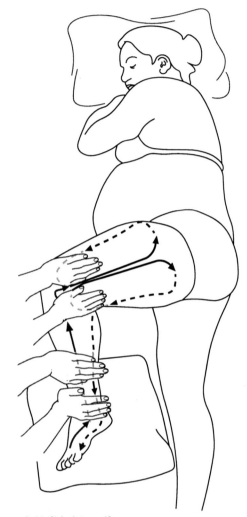

Figure 2.66. Side-lying effleurage up a bent leg.

someone in a side-lying position because the leg is not straight. Because of this, your effleurage must turn a corner on the way up and down the leg. I do about three effleurages and after the fourth trip up the leg, I stay at the hip for overhanded palmar kneading.

2. **Overhanded palmar kneading to the hip**: Side-lying is ideal for overhanded palmar kneading to the hip because the whole area, including the gluteals, is exposed and easily accessible.

Stand back from the hip and lean toward it with a stride posture. Use the same direction of pressure: toward the heart with each stroke pushing up and out, with one hand following the other hand around and around the whole gluteal muscle mass. Check in about pressure as this is the place where the mom can sometimes take additional pressure. Use a slow and steady rhythm.

I use this stroke to prepare the area for the more specific massage strokes, again working from general, big strokes like this one to nitty-gritty, small and focused strokes. Overhanded palmar kneading is also used to open up circulation to the lower extremity at the hip. You can also alternate from overhanded palmar kneading to reinforced palmar kneading and then back to overhanded palmar kneading again.

3. **Alternate thumb kneading to the hip**: Now that the surface tension is loosened and the area is warmed up, you can start to work deeper. Use alternate thumb kneading all around the head of the femur, including the gluteal muscles. Concentrate on massaging the attachment points of these muscles at the iliac crest and the ischial tuberosity, where the hamstrings attach from the back of the thigh. Be sure to be on the tips of your thumbs and move slowly for greater pressure. Use alternate thumb kneading liberally all around the hip.

4. **Reinforced fingertip kneading to the hip**: With the fingertips of one hand stacked on the other, knead the whole hip area. This stroke is very penetrating, so go easy with the first round and pick up the pressure as you continue to massage. The side-lying posture exposes more tender spots than face-up or face-down postures, so trigger points and other sore spots are easy to find.

5. **Overhanded palmar kneading to the hip**: To smooth over the picky and penetrating previous strokes, begin to back out to more general strokes with overhanded palmar kneading to the hip. Throw in an effleurage to connect what you are doing at the hip to what you are going to do on the rest of the leg, starting with the upper leg and thigh.

6. **Wringing to the thigh with a focus on the iliotibial band**: Wring across the iliotibial band, including the hamstrings on the back of the thigh and quadriceps on the front. With the mom in side-lying, stand facing her and lean in the stride position with your arms outstretched toward the leg. Wrap your hands around the thigh and wring across the iliotibial band, reaching all the way across the quadriceps to the adductors on the front and across the hamstrings to the adductors from the back.

Switch from this big-handed wringing to a smaller thumb wringing by putting your hands in a wrap around position so just the thumbs push and pull across the iliotibial structure. The fingers on the back of the thigh and the fingers on the front can make sure the hamstrings and quadriceps get a workout even as the thumbs focus in on the iliotibial band.

Travel up and down the outside of the thigh with thumb wringing at least three or four times. Be sure to get the full length of the iliotibial band, right to the tibial attachment at the knee.

7. **Alternate thumb kneading to the quadriceps**: Stand facing the mom's head. Massage the front of the thigh with alternate thumb kneading going up and down in the direction of the muscle fibers. You can also do some kneading across the fibers.

8. **Wringing to the thigh**: After alternate thumb kneading to the thigh, you may want to back out to wringing again for its eraser effect on the quadriceps. Again, the idea is to work with your massage from general strokes to specific strokes and then back out to general strokes again.

The whole thigh may be very tender to the touch, with swelling making the tissues strained with extra tension. Wringing is always great to break up any surface tension in this part of the body that is carrying extra weight or swelling as the baby gets bigger.

9. **Thumb compression to the iliotibial band.** Use both kinds: the poke-and-press variety

(digital compression) and then the trigger-point work with breathing and concentration. I use thumb compression along the iliotibial band, working about three trigger points and lots of poke and press everywhere.

10. **Wringing up and down the leg from hip to toes**: This wringing links the upper- and lower-leg massages. In the lower half of the leg, the wringing is preparatory and in the upper half of the leg, it is now finishing. Be sure to ask the mom how much of this stroke she would like: "Should I do this a little firmer? A little longer?"

11. **Alternate thumb kneading to the lower leg**: With my partner in the side-lying position, I employ the same routine of strokes that I use when my patient is face up (or down). But the beauty of the side-lying position is that the lower leg is so nicely exposed, front and back. If you need to, you can easily work both the gastrocnemius muscle in the back of the calf, as well as the tibialis anterior on the front. Use alternate thumb kneading all along the tibialis anterior from just below the knee to the base of the big toe. The tibialis anterior is just to the outside of the ridge of the tibia. Make your alternate thumb kneading tiny and powerful, especially as you move to the foot itself and along the tibialis anterior to the inside aspect of the arch.

Transition: Wring from the calf to the ankles and feet to bridge the lower leg massage to the foot massage.

FEET AND ANKLES (SIDE-LYING)

You can use the same strokes for the side-lying foot massage that you used in the first trimester, just adjusting to suit the new position.

1. **Wringing to the whole foot**: Wring from the ankle to the toes and back.

2. **Kneading to the ankles**: Knead around the ankle bones with your thumbs. You will need to hold the foot in your hands so it is slightly elevated and your hands can work freely.

3. **Alternate thumb kneading to the top of the foot** (3x or more).

4. **Corkscrew the toes.**

5. **Wringing to the whole foot**: Include the top of the foot and the sole (3x).

6. **Thumb wringing to the sole**: Use your thumbs to wring the sole of the foot any way you can (3x).

7. **Alternate thumb kneading to the sole** (3x).

8. **Wringing to finish**: Wringing to the foot, going slower and slower until you finish.

The increasing weight of the baby and pressure against the pelvic floor, with circulatory obstruction to the lower extremities, makes a foot massage an essential part of the second trimester massage. Both alternate thumb kneading and toe wringing are sure favorites.

When my daughter was in her second trimester, her feet became her favorite place to get massaged. When she was a kid, she would remember if I "missed" a toe in my weekly Wednesday family massage. In her second trimester pregnancy massages, she insisted that I should be just as thorough with the toe wringing and add another set of twisters to the mix. I always advocate three times for every stroke throughout the full-body massage, but with Crystal I lost count of the number of toe-massage rotations!

ARMS, HEAD, AND NECK (SIDE-LYING)

Arms are easy to massage in side-lying position—an easier adaptation than the leg massage in side-lying. With my patient in side-lying position, I massage the arm on top first, and when my patient turns to the other side, I massage the other arm.

If the mom cannot switch sides, then you can still massage the lower side of the body with a few adaptations. Use the "under the body" technique of levering up into the body from the table or massage surface. Do the best you can to balance your treatment on both sides of the mom's body.

Head and neck massages are easily adapted to side-lying position. In fact, the neck is *more* accessible in side-lying than in supine because you can get both hands on the neck for alternate thumb kneading, fingertip kneading, and alternating digital compression to the occipital ridge.

Third Trimester Massage

The third trimester pregnancy massage is generally the same as the progression of massages from first and second trimesters but with more serious prep for delivery as the trimester closes. Now that the mom is at her highest weight and her body is under the most pressure, she will likely have many pregnancy symptoms and your massages will have the biggest benefit. If you haven't done so already, include hydrotherapy in your massage, with cold wraps for the breasts and lower legs.

Timing

I always do a sixty- to ninety-minute full-body massage through to the end of the third trimester. As much as possible, I include family members with as many tandem massage tutorials as possible.

Patient positioning

This last trimester of massages is usually done in the side-lying position, but if that is uncomfortable, you can use the face-down position described on page 27. At this stage of pregnancy, your mom might have to move a few times to stay comfortable for an hour-long massage, moving from side-lying to face down to side-lying again. I always prop my supine patient up on two or three pillows so her head and shoulders are elevated.

Massage for the third trimester

In the last trimester, massages will include full-body work as in the first two trimesters, with a few changes as discussed below. You may also need to supplement the basic full-body massage with massages to address special symptoms, such as flat feet. Chapter 3 discusses what to do for many of the most common symptoms. If you're starting your third trimester, you will also want to start practicing labor and delivery massages so you are prepared when the time comes. See chapter 4 for details.

The biggest change for massaging in this last trimester is in the elevation of the patient if she is face up. For example, in the photo on the cover of this book, not only are Sarah's legs elevated above the heart for good lower leg drainage and venous return (the legs can never be too high), but also the upper part of her body is raised so she can breathe easier. Although our cover girl doesn't look like her head is elevated, it is!

Other changes from the first two trimesters include the following:

- The mom may need to frequently change massage position due to changing discomfort and breathing issues.
- Add more practice for labor, with counterpressure on the sacrum and verbal coaching for breathing and letting go of tension. Detailed instructions for this technique are included on page 59. Practice, practice, practice!
- Pay more attention to the inner thigh and low back.
- Introduce cold breast wraps as a warm-up for breastfeeding.
- Spend more time on your breast massage routine.
- Build a bigger massage team. Get everyone practicing counterpressure pain management routines.
- Practice a care for the caregiver routine, with head, neck, and shoulder massage to help build endurance for massaging long hours in preparation for labor and delivery.

Third trimester massage specialties

BREASTS

Breast massages should be longer, with more attention to the attachments of the pectoralis muscles to the sternum and armpit. Including the entire armpit in your breast massage stimulates the vascular and lymphatic systems. You can do this with a long scooping stroke from the upper area of the armpit toward the nipple. Do lots of massage to the clavicle and the upper chest to keep this area open and resisting pressure from the growing breasts, which will encourage stooping shoulders and tight pectorals.

A diaphragm massage may be needed if the baby has not dropped yet. The mom may have trouble breathing as the baby presses against her diaphragm and restricts her ability to draw a full breath. Refer to the respiratory massages beginning on page 76 for help alleviating this discomfort.

ABDOMEN

Do lots of massage around the edges of the abdomen with additional oils for stretch mark prevention, especially on the lower parts of the abdomen where the most scarring occurs. I also focus on the digestive tract and include leg pumping and leg rotations that are a great help for constipation (page 79).

BACK

Throughout the third trimester, practice massages for the back with the mom in a seated position. You want to be practiced in case you need to use this position during labor. One position to try has the mom sitting on the edge of the bed, with you in a shiatsu posture behind her. Run through the whole back massage sequence to see how you can adapt your strokes.

Massaging the mom while she is standing is the last posture to get good at in preparation for labor. Some women want to walk the hall and never sit down, let alone lie down. Lots of standing births are happening in western countries now as they have been happening for years in countries all over the world. Our hospitals accommodate all manner of deliveries, so practice these seemingly unusual postures to administer massage.

LEGS AND FEET

Elevate the legs for your leg massages. You will need to adjust your posture to accommodate the height of the legs.

Add cold footbaths (page 31) before and after foot massages.

The inner thighs and perineal area deserve an increasing focus of attention as the due date approaches. Some ideas for preparation of this key birthing area are as follows:

- Use hot water bottles to warm the adductors before and after working on the inner thigh. The mom can "hatch" the hot water bottle while sitting.
- Use lots of wringing from the top of the thigh to the knee while the mom is in a supine position, as she may be for baby delivery.
- Use alternate thumb kneading on the quadriceps and the adductors from high on the leg all the way down to the knee. The knees are now carrying more weight than they have ever carried before. Be sure to focus some kneading where the four quadriceps muscles come together at the patellar tendon at the knee (see Figure 2.19). Use tiny, firm alternate thumb kneading down to the attachment of the tendon to the tibia. Use open-handed alternate thumb kneading around the patella.
- Include single-handed fingertip kneading to the adductors as part of your leg routine. Pay particular attention to the attachments of the muscles at the pubic bone all the way down to the knee. You can feel the attachment points with your fingers, but Figure 2.17 will also guide you. Move slowly because these attachments are often tender to the touch.

"My experience with massage started out as recreational, the kind you have at the spa. When I got pregnant, they became more of a therapeutic experience and honestly became quite essential the later into the pregnancy I got. I was introduced to Christine in the beginning of my second trimester and we began seeing each other regularly. Eventually Christine recruited my husband into the massage experience. He seemed to pick it up easily. He works with his hands as a joiner; I think his finesse at work with the fine lines and grains of wood allowed him to quickly find all my trouble spots. The time we spent together exchanging massage was really intimate and seemed to help him be more part of the pregnancy experience. Christine also taught my mother how to do pregnancy massage. My mom is a master typist and has experience in nursing, so she too seemed to pick up massage skill quite quickly. Towards the last month of my pregnancy, I began to experience high blood pressure. The nurses and midwives I had been seeing encouraged me to visit the hospital for checkups every couple days. During the days I didn't go to the hospital, I had a massage to help control my blood pressure. The massages helped hold off delivery for two more weeks, which allowed my baby more time in the womb so she wouldn't be premature.

My water broke in the early morning and I ended up going to the hospital right away to have some monitoring done because of my blood pressure problem. I was eventually induced around 11:30 am and began to have contractions very shortly after that. Darren, my mom, and the nurses all spent time doing counterpressure on my low back during contractions. They used the palms of their hands with very intense (by my request) pressure. Everyone had sore, shaky arms later due to how much pressure I wanted through each contraction. When Christine arrived that evening, my legs were shaking from being on all fours or standing and bending over the bed through the contractions. It was like I had no control over my legs—they were just vibrating even while I was relaxing. My mom and Christine began working on my legs and my husband

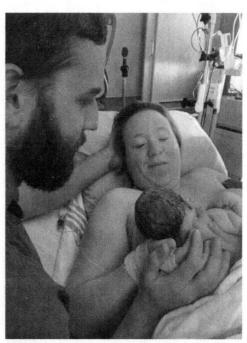

Figure 2.67. Fallon and Darren are one of my favorite couples. Darren was amazing in how quickly he picked up the massage strokes.

coached me through breathing techniques, sometimes even reminding me to breathe. When it came time to push, Christine and my mom were at my legs, holding them in place as I pushed, my husband coaching me through each one. Forty-five minutes later, at 00:03 on October 24, 2017, our baby girl entered the world.

Massage definitely helped throughout the pregnancy and labor and delivery, but it was for the pain after birth, the sore muscles and the back pain, that massage really came in handy. Even weeks later, when I was feeling much better physically, breastfeeding and even just carrying the wee one (who was light) got to me in ways I didn't expect. So when I got my massages after the delivery and the following weeks, I was looking so forward to them and felt that I needed them." —Fallon

Massage Treatments for Specific Maternity Conditions

This chapter outlines specific treatments of some of the most common conditions of pregnancy that are treatable with massage and various forms of hydrotherapy. Hydrotherapy uses water to treat a variety of conditions. In pregnancy, hydrotherapy treatments range from cold breast wraps, contrast temperature baths, and Epsom salt baths.

The main factor at play here is the baby's growth and the effect this has on the mother's body. The baby's growth creates a short-term imbalance, making the rest of the body shift around to accommodate the changes. These shifts can cause many problems, such as knee pain, flat feet, and trouble breathing. Some conditions might completely disappear after the delivery, but others can linger. Massage can provide immediate relief during the pregnancy and help prevent long-term effects.

The conditions are discussed as I travel from the top of the body to the bottom, nose to toes, starting with headaches and sore neck, moving on to carpal tunnel syndrome and difficulty breathing, and then through all the many conditions that affect the lower body during pregnancy.

An important caution: massage treatments for some of the complex conditions discussed in this chapter will be most effective and safest in the hands of a professional massage therapist. A registered massage therapist is well-trained in the latest contraindications and can be a guide to the best ways to approach safe massaging. I urge moms with persistent symptoms to seek appropriate professional help as soon as possible (medical, midwifery, nursing, and other allied health professionals, including professional massage therapy). This is not to discount your own massage contributions to the mom's well-being, but don't hesitate to seek professional help when needed.

Quick Guide to Specific Massage Treatments

Upper Extremities		*Lower Extremities*	
Headaches	66	Hip problems	85
Care for the caregivers (in-chair neck and shoulder massage)	67	Sciatica	85
		Contracted iliotibial band	86
Neck and shoulder problems	71	Knee problems	88
Carpal tunnel syndrome	73	Varicose veins	88
		Leg cramping	90
Trunk of the Body		Shin splints	91
Nausea and morning sickness (digestive)	75	Flat feet	92
Respiratory problems	75		
Constipation	78		
Spinal problems	80		

Upper Extremities

In pregnancy, the most frequent problems for the upper extremities are headaches and arm and hand pain.

Headaches

Many prenatal headaches are caused by changing shoulder and neck pressure due to growing breasts. Even pain across the forehead or temples is often referred pain from tension in the neck. Such headaches are often relieved when tension in the neck is alleviated and circulation to the head is improved. Always start a headache treatment by massaging the neck as the most likely cause of headaches. Self-massage is useful here. People with a headache often do what comes naturally by reaching up and massaging their neck with one hand or the other.

Symptoms in the head can also stem from upper-respiratory problems such as sinus congestion and allergies, so opening the sinuses above and below the eye will give relief. Facial stroking from the midline of the face to the outer aspects can often relieve a headache, especially a sinus headache.

Fluid retention, especially in the second and third trimesters, can be experienced not only in the arms and legs, but also in the head (as the fifth extremity). Often, as the swelling is addressed through massage of the extremities, headaches also diminish.

Other headaches result from hormonal changes. These can also be helped with massage.

The worst headache I ever treated was in a huge hospital in Guatemala City in a unit of nothing but C-section deliveries. I came across a woman sitting in her hospital gown in a crowded hallway waiting for a bed. She had had a spinal injection for her C-section and the resulting headache was nauseating, one of the worst I'd ever seen. It was as though she was having an allergic reaction to the procedure. I seized the opportunity to teach the woman's family and other hospital workers to give a shoulder and neck massage. In just twenty minutes, she went from crying to smiling. By the time they found her a bed, her headache was gone. The unit was full of women with similar headaches, so soon I was being called over from all directions! After returning to Canada, my medical colleagues informed me that the headaches were likely caused by poorly administered epidurals.

Light headaches caused by stress or lack of sleep are often helped by massaging the temples and the occipital ridge at the back of the head and base of the skull. The temples are easily massaged with stiff fingertip kneading at the hypersensitive area right on the hairline where the skin and scalp meet. More serious headaches need a good grip at the back of the head at the top of the spine. When I'm massaging someone who is sitting in a chair, I use the web between my thumb and fingers to cup at the bottom of the occipital ridge and pull up gently to lengthen the spine.

Cold water footbaths (see page 31) can be an effective headache treatment. The body sees the cold footbath as a "counterirritant" and goes looking to address the issue at the feet, giving the head a neurological rest. This isn't a perfect treatment of all headaches, but it works well for many, combined with your relieving massage treatment, of course!

RELIEVING NECK TENSION TO RELIEVE HEADACHES

When I am treating someone lying supine, I hold the head along the base of the skull, pulling the head toward me with steady pressure (traction). I then pull up into the occipital ridge of the skull, on one side of that ridge only, so the face rotates to the side. I then do the traction on the other side, and the head gently rolls the other way. The action of the head passively rolling relaxes the neck and often makes cranial tension disappear. It usually only takes a few minutes of neck massage for discomfort to lessen.

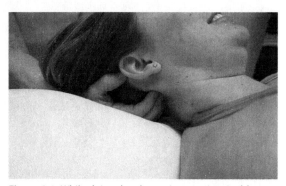

Figure 3.1. While doing the alternating traction, I add in some fingertip kneading to those tight muscle attachments at the base of the skull at the occipital ridge. The combination of traction and massage works wonders. This is one of my patients' favorite massage routines.

CARE FOR THE CAREGIVERS (IN-CHAIR NECK AND SHOULDER MASSAGE)

This "kitchen table" head, neck, and shoulder massage is great for headaches and as care for birthing partners. This massage is adaptable for sitting at the kitchen table, while watching television, or on the back porch.

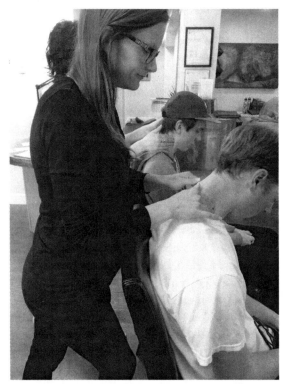

Figure 3.2. I teach this in-chair massage in my pregnancy massage classes, with partners sitting in front of the pregnant mom while she practices.

Use your partner's feedback as your guide. For example, you might spend more time around the eyes or temples or jaw if that seems to be the area that elicits the most relief. Look for differences between different people's shoulders and look for differences between left and right sides of the same individual. Have your partner remove his or her eyeglasses and lean forward against a table with a pillow or two to rest the arms or elbows on. Stand close by your partner's side or back to begin. If you need to review the location of the upper back and shoulder muscles, see Figure 2.1.

1. **Natural squeeze to the shoulders and arms:** Place both hands on the shoulders and give a squeeze to develop a rapport and accustom the person to your touch. Work down the arm, alternately squeezing and releasing.

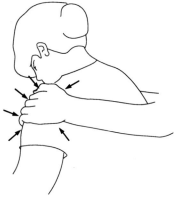

Figure 3.3. Starting at the shoulder and working down the arm, squeeze and release the muscles as a warm-up for your hands and to "pass the PPT." P = posture. Do you have the right posture to get good pressure and protect your back? P = pressure. Ask your partner if you should give more or less pressure. T = test.

2. **Scoop the trapezius:** Develop the squeeze, giving scoops of the trapezius with the heels of your hands. Lift the shoulder muscle up like a mother cat lifts up her kittens. Hold the muscle, coaching your partner through a couple of deep breaths, and then let go of the muscle on the last out breath. (Figure 3.4) This is my pressure gauge stroke. Be sure to ask for the F-word (feedback), using questions such as "Can I be firmer? Should I be lighter?"

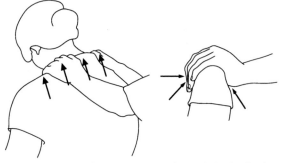

Figure 3.4. Scoop the trapezius muscles with the heels of your hands in a lifting action. Hold the muscle for a few breaths, and then let go.

3. **Digital compression on the rhomboids:**
   Move from the trapezius squeeze to digital compression with your thumbs. Position your thumbs on either side of the spine just under the occipital ridge. Taking care not to squeeze the throat with your fingers, and alternating between your thumbs as you work, poke and press, like walking with the tips of your thumbs on either side of the spine on the erector spinae from the occipital ridge until you get to the top of the rhomboids. Once you get to the rhomboids, slow down and work your static digital compression deeply until the bottom of the scapula. This area can be quite tight. Be sure to check with your partner that your pressure is right. Keep your thumbs at the same speed and rhythm as they alternate to work down both sides of the body. (Figure 3.5)

4. **Head tilts:** Always keep the nose pointing forward during this sequence. Have your partner sit up. Move to your partner's side

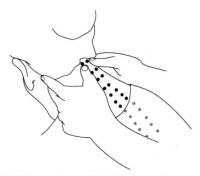

Figure 3.5. Poke and press. The thumbs do the work.

and place one hand on the forehead and one at the base of the skull using the web of your hand between the thumb and fingers. Lift and slowly tilt the head three times in each direction, pivoting the head on the top of the spine. Be sure your movements are slow and careful. Sometimes I use these head tilts at the start of a headache treatment to see how stiff the person's neck is since this is a common origin of headaches.

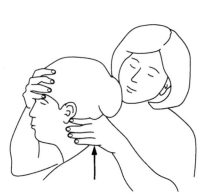

a. With a scooping action, lift at the back of the head under the occipital ridge to give traction.

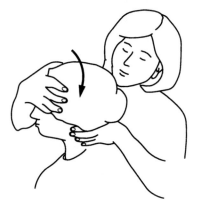

b. Gently move ear to shoulder.

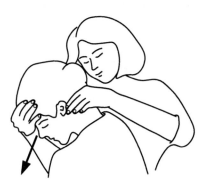

c. Drop the chin to chest.

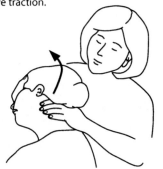

d. Gently move ear to opposite shoulder.

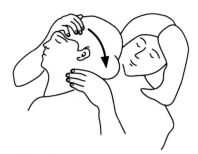

e. Tilt head backward.

Figure 3.6. Head tilts. Secure the head by placing one hand on the forehead. (Be careful not to cover up the eyes.) With the other hand in an open C-shape, lift up against the base of the skull in a slight traction motion.

5. **Temporal kneading**: Move to the back of your partner and place your fingertips on the temples right at the hairline. Slowly knead all around the temple and the jaw joint area. Have the person release his or her jaw by relaxing the mouth open slightly.

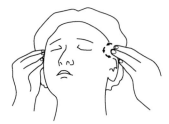

Figure 3.7. Temporal kneading.

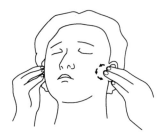

Figure 3.8. Temporal mandibular kneading on the chin bone in front of the bottom of the ears.

6. **Percussive tapotement for the upper back**: For the trapezius, deltoids, and rhomboids, give a percussive tapotement massage. (See pages 21–24 for a description of how to do these strokes.)
   - Loose fingertip hacking
   - Stiff-fingered hacking
   - Cupping
   - Beating
   - Pounding

7. **Percussive tapotement for the lower back**: Have your partner lean forward again, placing elbows on the knees and dropping the head down. Stand to the side and perform this percussion over the rest of the back, being careful not to thump on the spine itself.

8. **Shoulder squeeze (repeat)**.

9. **Head tilts (repeat)**.

10. **Light reflex stroking**: Stroke lightly with your fingertips from the top of the head and out to the shoulders and arms and from the top of

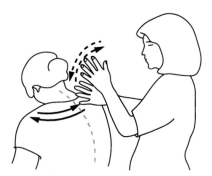

a. Loose fingertip hacking (flicking)

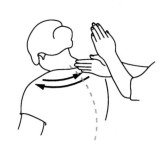

b. Stiff fingertip hacking (chopping)

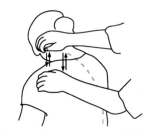

c. Cupping (Be sure you get a hollow sound, not a slapping sound.)

Figure 3.9. Percussive tapotement.

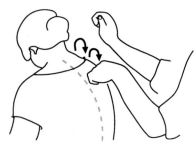

d. Beating (monkey paw with a flip-flop wrist)

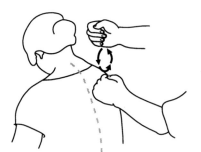

e. Pounding (Roll your fists toward your body in a Ferris wheel.)

the head down the spine. Be sure not to end with a whack on the back and hearty "Now it's my turn!" or "Up and at 'em!"

Neck and shoulder problems

Every woman will have bigger breasts by the second and third trimesters, which will cause a change in the dynamic tension of the head, neck, and shoulders. Focusing your massage on the neck and shoulders with lots of fingertip kneading and palmar scooping to the trapezius muscles (Figure 3.4) will help relieve this growing problem.

You can also practice neck and shoulder massages during the second and third trimesters in preparation for postpartum breastfeeding and the muscular aches and pains associated with it.

The following massage strokes (Figures 3.10 to 3.18) are all with the mom on her back. The head is rotated or stretched (ear to shoulder) when necessary to accommodate strokes along the side of the neck.

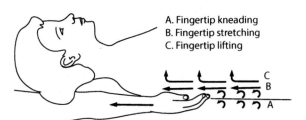

A. Fingertip kneading
B. Fingertip stretching
C. Fingertip lifting

Figure 3.10. Slide your hands as far as possible under the mom's back and lever up. You can give a surprisingly effective massage in this position.

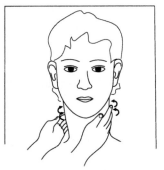

Figure 3.13. Bilateral fingertip kneading to the sides of the neck up to the base of the skull.

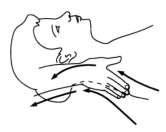

Figure 3.11. Reflex stroking to the neck muscles.

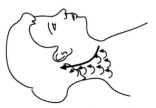

Figure 3.14. Deep fingertip kneading to the trapezius and neck muscles up to the base of the skull.

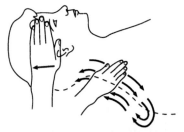

Figure 3.12. Modified effleurage to the neck. Use one hand to press the head gently to the side to give a little more space for the effleurage.

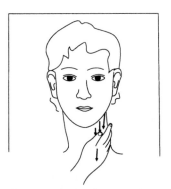

Figure 3.15. Light finger stroking with pressure from the head down. This stroke can help with lymphatic drainage.

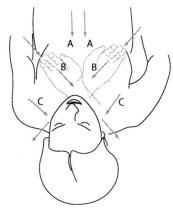

Figure 3.16. Scooping to the rhomboids, erector spinae, and trapezius. Slide your hands under the mom's body and scoop them toward you to work the erector spinae (A), rhomboids (B), and trapezius muscles (C). Alternate your hands scooping diagonally across the mom's back as you pull toward you. Be sure to avoid any pressure on the spinal column itself.

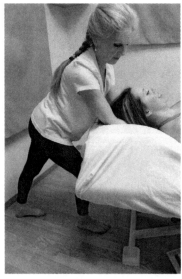

Figure 3.17. To get your body in the right position for this scooping stroke, be sure to use the stride position.

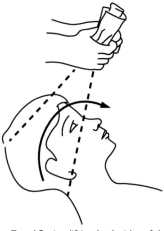

a. Towel flexion lifting both sides of the towel together

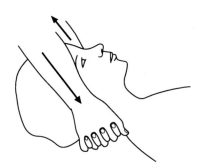

b. Interlocked hands under the occipital ridge

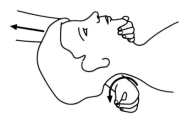

c. With one hand under the chin, pull toward you while the other hand rolls under the occipital ridge.

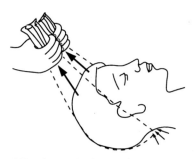

d. Towel extension (traction)

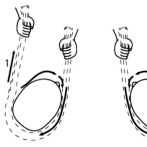

e. Face rolls by pulling straight up on one side of the towel and then the other, so the head gently rotates from side to side

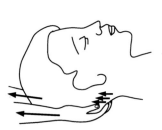

f. Fingertip traction from the occipital ridge

Figure 3.18. Methods to work tension out of the neck.

Carpal tunnel syndrome

Carpal tunnel syndrome is caused by a pinching of the median nerve, which runs from the neck down the arm to the hand. It causes pain, numbness, or tingling in the wrist and hand where the nerve supplies the sensations for the half of the hand that houses the middle finger, pointer finger, and thumb.

Most women experiencing this painful condition have used their hands in some significant way, such as stained-glass artists, knitters, and upper-arm athletes like tennis and squash players. Avid texters and computer workers are also frequent victims of carpal tunnel syndrome.

In pregnancy, carpal tunnel syndrome is often caused by swelling. The swelling of the body, especially in the hands, causes the carpal bones of the wrist to get jammed together, pinching the median nerve. This results in a variety of problems, such as not being able to wear rings or not being able to pick things up or have a strong, confident grip.

Carpal tunnel syndrome, when severe, is usually treated by splinting the wrists overnight. One of my first pregnant patients had such severe carpal tunnel syndrome that she was wearing splints 24/7. (And this was before computers!) I brought her into my massage class for a massage therapy case study. She was massaged on a regular basis for the last month of her pregnancy and for the first month of her postpartum with great results. With a daily application of massage, she was able to immediately hold her newborn baby securely, without the aid of splints.

Although discomfort is felt primarily in the wrists, massage helps to diminish pain and restore circulation by reducing edema (swelling) throughout the entire arm.

First massage the head, neck, and shoulders to open up circulation to the arm. People with rounded shoulders can have tight muscles that clamp down on the median nerve where it exits from the neck vertebrae. A squeezing of the nerve anywhere along its route gives rise to pain farther along the arm. Sometimes simply loosening up the top of the arm and neck area will help dissipate the problem. Use firm pressure with all your strokes to work the tension out of the shoulders. Doing the backstroke in the pool can also help loosen up this area.

Then move to an arm and hand massage. Use our basic routine for the arm (pages 43–47). For all strokes, use firm pressure and small strokes, especially at the wrist, on the palm, and for each individual finger. I spend a lot of time from the elbow down, reducing swelling by pushing my thumbs in short upward strokes, alternating with a mini-effleurage in between.

As I work on the forearm with thumb and palmar kneading, I move the hand slowly between flexion and extension. This stretching movement maximizes effectiveness of the therapeutic strokes.

You may also want to add in hydrotherapy contrast (cold and warm) arm bathing.

Some women have very swollen arms in the second and third trimesters and never experience carpal tunnel syndrome. Other women have carpal tunnel syndrome in the last weeks and months of pregnancy, and yet do not have significant swelling. I find each patient distinctly different in the nature of her symptoms, which can range from complete numbness to partial tingling. The treatment is still basically the same. Work the head, neck, and shoulder area and then down the arm to the wrist and hand. Find the person's particular areas of tension and work toward developing a treatment plan that yields the best results.

The more you can loosen up the head, neck, and shoulders and work the elbow, the better the hand feels. Lessening the pressure and edema in the arms, even if it is just for a few hours, gives a feeling of relief and ease of movement. This condition is like a headache in the arm, but one that for some people doesn't go away. The massage routine outlined above can be done several times each day for at least twenty minutes each time (minimum ten minutes per arm).

The best times for massaging anybody with carpal tunnel syndrome or just swelling in the arms

MASSAGE MENU FOR CARPAL TUNNEL SYNDROME

START WITH THE ARM:

1. **Effleurage:** Apply deep, slow effleurage from the hand to the shoulder, with pressure only on the up stroke.

2. **Palmar kneading to the upper arm and deltoid:** Use deep, slow strokes.

3. **Alternate thumb kneading to the upper arm:** Use alternate thumb kneading on the deltoid, the biceps, the triceps. Knead the inner elbow at least six times.

4. **Wringing to the forearm:** With open-handed, C-shaped hands, wring from the inner elbow down the forearm and back up to the elbow.

5. **Effleurage to the forearm:** Use deep, slow effleurage from the wrist up to the elbow. Ask the mom if your pressure should be firmer or softer.

6. **Thumb kneading to the forearm:** If there is muscle definition in the forearm, follow the contours of the muscles with your thumb strokes, keeping them penetrating and deep.

7. **Palmar kneading to the forearm:** Use the flat of your hand to smooth out the deep, grooving thumb kneading with similarly deep palmar kneading strokes.

8. **Frictioning:** Apply frictioning to any knotted or sensitive areas with fingertips, thumbs, or ice. Use ice frictioning liberally.

9. **Wringing to the forearm:** Move up and down with the stroke at least three times (but you can never do too much wringing).

10. **Repeat steps 6 to 9:** (3x).

MOVE TO THE HAND:

11. **Digital compression to palm:** Move slowly and firmly. Focus on the heel of the hand, where the muscles may be pinching the nerve.

12. **Thumb stroking to palm:** Use deep thumb stroking to the palm of the hand in all directions (up and down and across) to stretch out the palmar fascia.

13. **Corkscrew the fingers:** Pay special attention to the base of the fingers.

14. **Alternate thumb kneading to palm:** Holding wrist bent back, alternate thumb knead the palm of the hands with special attention to the wrist bones. Use very small and focused strokes.

15. **Alternate thumb kneading to the back of the wrist:** Holding the forearm up with the wrist bent down, do alternate thumb kneading to the top of the carpal bones at the wrist (again using small, focused, and firm strokes).

16. **Thumb stroking to forearm:** Using short, deep, slow thumb strokes, move from the base of the hand halfway up the forearm. Make the strokes shorter and more concentrated near the wrist. Ask the mom for feedback about her tolerance for the pressure of this stroke.

17. **Finish:** Finish with wringing and then effleurage to the whole arm, followed by light reflex stroking.

are last thing at night and first thing in the morning. At the end of the day, people's arms are swollen due to gravity. A similar problem occurs at night, during which there is no movement of the arms while someone is sleeping. Massaging first thing in the morning helps get the circulation moving and relieves any pain or swelling that may have built up during the night.

This condition can sometimes be treated with self-massage since the mom can easily access the areas of treatment. Self-massage to the forearm, especially with ice frictioning to the wrist three times a day, can be highly effective. Usually the symptoms are worse on one hand than the other, but if both the mom's hands are in pain, she won't be able to apply adequate pressure for self-massage. In that case, everyone else needs to get really good at providing her with massage relief.

Trunk of the Body

Conditions affecting the trunk of the body during pregnancy most often include respiratory complaints, such as trouble breathing, and digestive problems such as constipation.

Use your general massage for the back (pages 34–35 and 56–60) to help the nerves run smoothly out of the spine to the organs. The nerves that exit from the thoracic area (upper and middle back) work the lungs, and the nerves from the lumbar area (low back) work the digestive system. So massage the back thoroughly, knowing that you are helping the frontal problems such as digestive and respiratory dysfunction.

Nausea and morning sickness (digestive)

For nausea and morning sickness, a combination of respiratory and digestive massage often works wonders. The back of the neck usually gets all the attention in massage, but massage for the front of the neck, involving the muscles of the throat, can be an effective treatment of nausea. The throat and soft palate under the chin are the intersection of the digestive and respiratory conditions, sharing a common passageway for both breathing and eating. Not surprisingly, the massage strokes for treating nausea also work to open up breathing.

1. **Light stroking to front of neck**: Start with light reflex stroking for the front of the neck all the way down the route of the digestive system to the abdomen. Even just this light stroking can be soothing, often easing feelings of nausea.

2. **Scooping to the throat**: With one hand, scoop down the front of the throat, working from the soft palate to the sternum.

3. **Fingertip kneading to the sternocleidomastoid muscles**: Kneading the sternocleidomastoid muscles that run from the back of the neck down the sides to the front can ease tension in the front of the throat and make swallowing easier.

4. **Back of the neck**: Use dorsal scooping, towel work, traction, and fingertip kneading to the occipital ridge. See pages 71–72. All will increase the ease of movement and circulatory flow from the head to the trunk of the body.

5. **Kneading and stroking from the mouth to the abdomen**: Palmar stroking, fingertip stroking, and all of the kneading strokes can be applied from the mouth to the stomach, especially along the clavicle and down the sternum.

6. **Abdominal massage**: Include an abdominal massage (pages 47–49) to finish up an antinausea treatment.

Respiratory problems

Respiratory massage during pregnancy is usually one of two types. One is to help alleviate the sinus congestion anyone—pregnant or not pregnant—has with a cold or flu. Respiratory congestion can be particularly troublesome in pregnancy, especially if the mom wants to avoid taking any medications.

The second type of respiratory massage, more specific to pregnancy, helps the mom breathe easier in the second and third trimesters until the baby drops. As the baby grows in the second and third trimesters, it pushes up against the mom's ribs and diaphragm muscle, making it more difficult for her to comfortably draw a full breath of air. Before the baby drops in the last weeks of the pregnancy, you can help ease up the mom's breathing with diaphragmatic massage, rib raking, bilateral lifting, and upper chest massage. Rib raking becomes a popular stroke for better breathing.

No matter what kind of respiratory problem the mom has, your goal is to help her breathe better.

MASSAGE TO EASE BREATHING DUE TO CHEST OR SINUS CONGESTION

If the mom has chest congestion that makes breathing difficult, begin your massage with a steam bath, which will help loosen some of the mucus. Pour boiling water and a few drops of eucalyptus oil into a bowl. Have the mom sit in front of the bowl with her face in the vapor. Cover her head with a towel to make a steam tent and ask her to breathe slowly and deeply. Then apply cupping and other tapotement strokes to her back and chest to help her loosen up any congestion.

For upper respiratory congestion, shaking strokes to the nose and throat can also help ease

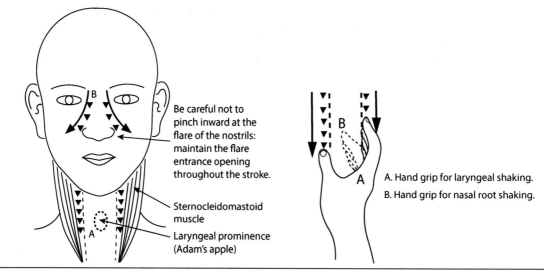

Figure 3.19. Respiratory shaking.

Be careful not to pinch inward at the flare of the nostrils: maintain the flare entrance opening throughout the stroke.

Sternocleidomastoid muscle

Laryngeal prominence (Adam's apple)

A. Hand grip for laryngeal shaking.

B. Hand grip for nasal root shaking.

breathing. For shaking strokes, make a C-shape with the hand and move your fingertips back and forth from side to side in a fast, but gentle fluttering motion. Use a large C-shape to fit the front of the neck and a smaller fingertip C-shape to run up and down the nose where it attaches to the face.

MASSAGE TO EASE BREATHING DUE TO THE BABY'S GROWTH

For breathing problems due to the baby's growth and position in the abdomen, a massage to the diaphragm and rib raking can ease breathing.

1. **Wringing to the trunk**: Start with wringing to both sides of the trunk of the body. You will have to jump over the pregnant tummy in the last trimesters, and that means the wringing will be best at the bottom of the chest before the big bump of the baby. Just adapt your strokes to glide over the baby and not squish anybody.

2. **Costal border scooping**: The sides of the mom are also a great place to ease up breathing with a scooping massage along the costal angle of the ribs. (Figure 3.21)

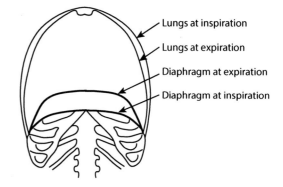

Lungs at inspiration

Lungs at expiration

Diaphragm at expiration

Diaphragm at inspiration

Figure 3.20. Basic structure of the lungs. The diaphragm muscle attaches to the ribs and goes through the body from the front to the back. It is like a big balloon sheath. That is why you can pop your ribs when you cough forcefully. As the baby gets larger, it can press against the diaphragm and ribs, causing much discomfort. Loosening the area up can make a little extra room for the mom to breathe with ease.

3. **Kneading and thumb stroking to the diaphragm**: Use fingertip kneading and bilateral thumb stretching to the attachments of the diaphragm to the ribs. (Figures 3.22 and 3.23) This is a great opportunity for family massage to encourage siblings to talk to the baby.

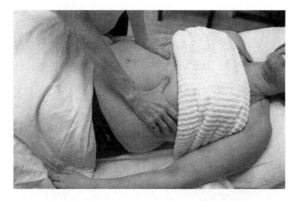

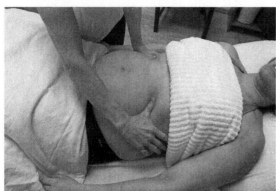

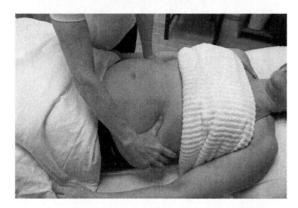

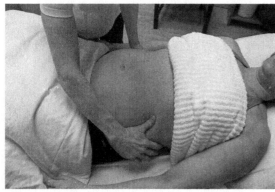

Figure 3.21. Costal border scooping.

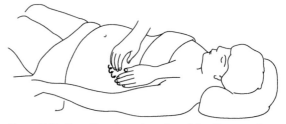

Figure 3.22. Kneading along the edge of the ribs may give some extra release to help breathing. Your fingers should roll over the edge of the costal angle (bottom rib) to get the diaphragm attachments.

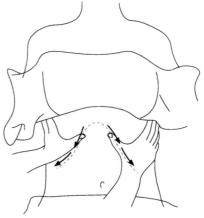

Figure 3.23. Bilateral thumb stretching under the costal angle.

4. **Overhanded rib raking**: Rib raking draws the fingers across the tiny intercostal muscles between the ribs to stretch them out to ease the mother's breathing when the baby is sitting high up against the ribs and diaphragm, causing shortness of breath.

A. Stand at the side of the table. Making a claw with your hand, reach across to the far side of the pregnant abdomen as far as you can and grip the ribs. Each fingertip of your "claw" should be between the ribs in the intercostal grooves.

B. Slowly lean back to pull up and around the trunk of the body following the diagonal direction of the ribs. Grip the intercostal muscles with slow, deep, continuous fingertip movements.

C. As one hand finishes the stroke, the next hand reaches over to the same start point. As one hand finishes the length of the stroke, the other hand begins. Do this until there is a significant change in breathing, usually after five to ten strokes.

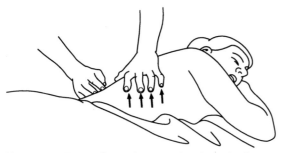

Figure 3.24. Fit your fingers between the ribs and pull to help stretch the intercostal muscles.

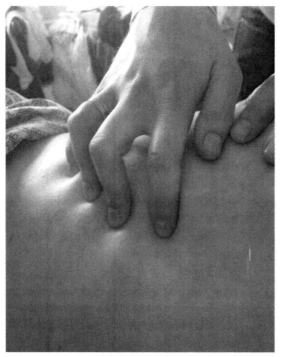

Figure 3.25. Use a claw-like hand for rib raking.

5. **Lifting to the abdomen**: Lifting strokes— either bilateral or overhanded—can also help ease breathing and relieve low back tension or pain.

- **Bilateral lifting**: Lean over the supine mom and circle your hands around to her back, your fingertips meeting at her spine. Then slowly, very slowly, lift up and pull toward the front, meeting at the top of the baby with very light contact to end the stroke and being careful to not squish the baby.

- **Overhanded lifting**: Work on one side of the mom and then the other, pulling toward yourself with alternating hands like you are bringing in an anchor off the side of a boat. Reach across the mom and tuck your hand under her back toward the spine. Then pull up toward you with the palm of your hand. As one hand finishes, the other should be starting. Walk around to the other side and do the same lifting on the other side of the mom's body. If you can't walk to the other side, it's possible to do both sides of the mom's body from one side. The lifting on the near side won't be "overhanded," but it will still balance both sides and relieve that low back pain/tension.

It is really important to practice rib raking and diaphragm massage during the second and third trimesters so that you are practiced in case these symptoms appear at the very end of the pregnancy in the final days, when the mom needs sleep the most!

Constipation

Digestive complaints can start early with daily heartburn. By the second and third trimesters, pregnant women often experience escalated and uncomfortable constipation. In the last couple weeks, when the baby drops, many women find they can breathe better, but the baby's pressure on the colon means constipation becomes a new problem. Aside from drinking the lake dry, hands-on massage will make a huge difference. Relieving constipation is very important so that hemorrhoids will not give rise to further discomfort in this stage of pregnancy, in labor and delivery, or in postpartum recovery.

Begin with the regular pregnancy abdominal massage routine (see page 47). Because of the obstruction of the growing child on the inside, you will need to adapt the strokes to focus more on the perimeter: the large intestine. Do your open C-shaped scooping from the top of the abdomen to the center and from the bottom to center in an alternating rhythm so the baby in the middle is not disturbed. The pressure of the stroke will be determined by how much room you have to maneuver. Sometimes I eliminate this stroke in the last trimester.

You can also again do lots of bilateral wringing and lifting, as you did for respiratory massage. Vibrations and fingertip kneading all around the large intestine will help with constipation and gas. Start where the small intestine hooks up to the large intestine on the lower right side of the abdomen. Follow the path of the digestive system, remembering to linger in the corners (flexures) of the large intestine. When you reach the lower left corner, you can glide across the bottom where the bladder is to start the circle again.

We instinctively do tapotement or percussive cupping to a baby's back once it has nursed to help it burp. You can use the same style of treatment of digestive complaints by working the low back with tapotement strokes.

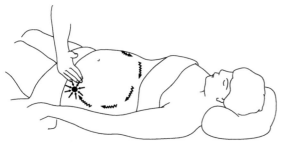

Figure 3.26. Vibrations and fingertip kneading along the path of the large intestine are effective treatments for constipation and gas. It is particularly useful to knead on the descending colon, especially on the lower left side of the abdomen.

LEG PUMPING

The most involved strokes for the maternity digestive system are movements, not massage strokes. Leg pumping is the best remedy for unwinding the digestive system. This is the same massage for treating babies with constipation or digestive complaints: abdominal massage, then leg pumping; abdominal massage, then leg pumping.

When a horse starts out of the barn, it lifts its tail and releases gas, feeling happier immediately. It needs activity to get its digestive and elimination systems working. Similarly, when people are immobilized, they also have compromised digestive systems. I teach abdominal massage, including the leg pumping, for people in wheelchairs to get digestion moving. This also works for anyone in a palliative condition. Leg pumping helps the hips give a peristaltic action to the contents of the large intestine, especially during the last weeks and days of the pregnancy when no one wants to move. There are three kinds of leg pumping I find most helpful to include before, during, and after an abdominal massage.

1. **Simultaneous leg pumping:** Hold the mom's legs with the knees supported by your hand or forearm while your other hand supports the feet. Bend both legs in toward her abdomen gently and firmly. To control the legs, keep them close together so they do not bend outward.

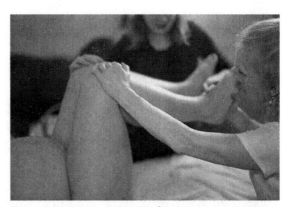

Figure 3.27. Using your hand or forearm to press against the knees will help you bend the mom's legs.

2. **Alternate leg pumping**: With the same hand grip, bend one leg at the knee, straight to the abdomen, and then straighten it out completely before bending the other knee. Do this at least ten times. In my tandem teaching tutorials, we each hold a leg and work as a team in the alternate leg pumping.

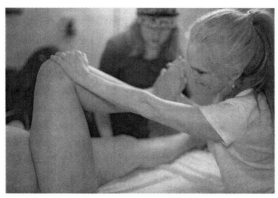

Figure 3.28. If you have a partner, each of you can support one leg. In that case, one hand can hold the bottom of the foot and the other hand can rest below the knee.

3. **Rotations**: Bend both legs up to the abdomen and then wrap your hands around the legs so they are snug against the mom's abdomen. Roll her lower body around in a circular movement, with the low back (lumbar area) getting a gentle massage. The low back is the source of nerves for the digestive area, so this massage is great stimulation for the digestive tract.

Do the three kinds of leg pumping for a few minutes. I recommend repeating this series of movements at least ten times, before the abdominal massage and after.

Spinal problems

We cannot leave the trunk of the body without addressing spinal issues. Some women have pre-existing back problems that become worse during the pregnancy. For example, if the woman has scoliosis (a lateral curve of the spine) whether it be a simple C-curve or a compound S-curve, that curve will take a great deal of pulling during the last trimesters.

You can try to mitigate the extra pressure on her spine with massage, working the muscles along the spine to stretch the contracted muscles and stimulate the overly stretched muscles to contract. Both contracted and stretched muscles need attention so they can recover from the daily strain of the back carrying more weight.

The more acute problems of kyphosis (humpback) and lordosis (swayback) often give rise to sacroiliac strain as the lumbar area gets pulled into a bigger lower-back curve. Kyphosis includes highly rounded shoulders, tight, shortened pectoral muscles, and stretched, weak back muscles; lordosis is an excessive curve of the spine at the low back.

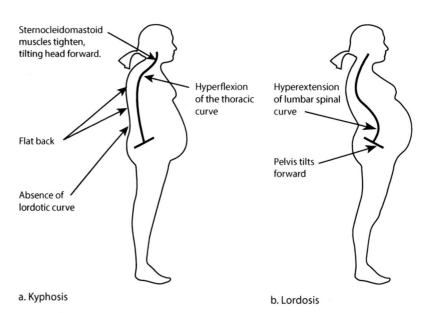

Sternocleidomastoid muscles tighten, tilting head forward.

Hyperflexion of the thoracic curve

Hyperextension of lumbar spinal curve

Flat back

Pelvis tilts forward

Absence of lordotic curve

a. Kyphosis

b. Lordosis

Figure 3.29. Conditions of kyphosis and lordosis can develop or become worse during pregnancy due to the weight of the breasts and growing abdomen.

As the pregnancy continues and the baby grows larger, these problems will escalate. As well as pain in the low back, the mom can have neck and shoulder pain as the body strains to move the head perpendicular to adapt to the curves in the back.

Daily massage is what works. First work with the mom in face-up position to stretch out the contracted pectoral muscles and then work with the mom face down or side-lying (both sides) to work on tightness and adhesions in the back muscles.

MASSAGE FOR KYPHOSIS AND LORDOSIS

Have the mom lie on her back with her arms raised and hands behind her head. See Figure 3.30 for towel positioning.

1. **Effleurage to the head, neck, shoulders, and abdomen.**

2. **Palmar stretching to the pectorals.** (Figures 3.31 to 3.34)

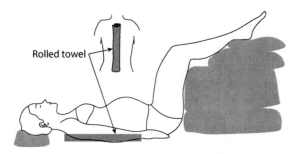

Figure 3.30. Corrective towel positioning for kyphosis and lordosis.

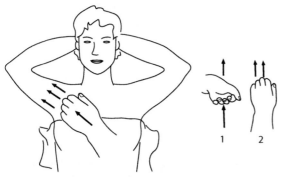

Figure 3.31. Stretch the pectoralis muscles with the backs of your fingers by rolling them across the muscle.

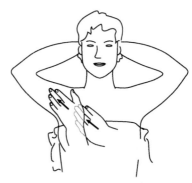

Figure 3.32. Overhanded palmar stretching pushing away from the pectoral attachment at the sternum (chest bone).

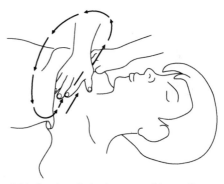

Figure 3.33. Overhanded palmar stretching pulling toward yourself.

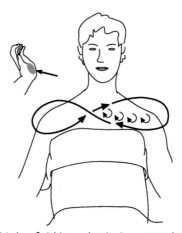

Figure 3.34. As a finishing or beginning pectoral stretch, use your palms to do a figure eight across the chest. Use the thenar eminence at the base of the thumb to knead circles around this path.

3. Thumb stretching to the pectorals.

4. **Frictioning to pressure points:** You can use your thumbs, fingertips, or palms. (Figure 3.35)

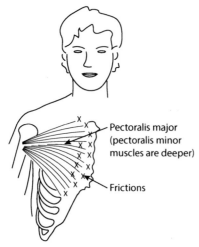

Figure 3.35. Friction points along the pectorals.

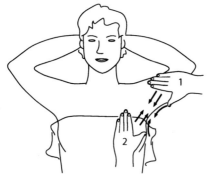

a. Axilla (armpit) scooping with the arm turned upward

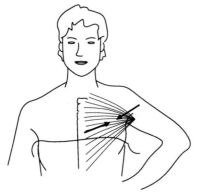

b. Scooping to the pectoralis major with the arm turned downward

Figure 3.36. Scooping to the lateral pectoral border with alternating hands.

5. Repeat palmar stretching/palmar kneading.

6. Scooping to pectorals. (Figure 3.36)

7. **Frictioning to the muscle attachments on the sternum.**

8. **Lymphatic drainage to the armpit:** Apply scooping strokes.

9. **Abdominal massage.**

10. **Neck twist.** (Figure 3.37)

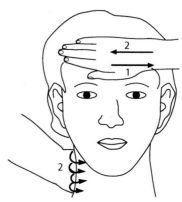

Figure 3.37. The neck twist is like a type of wringing. With one hand on the forehead and one reaching over the mom's body to the far side of the neck, lift the neck and pull the head so the face rotates toward you. As you push the face away from you, lift up from behind the neck and rotate it toward you to create a therapeutic stretching and elongation of the upper trapezius muscle.

11. **Thumb kneading to the sternocleidomastoid muscles.**

12. **Frictioning to the sternocleidomastoid muscles.**

13. **Finish:** Kneading, wringing, and effleurage.

14. **Prone back massage:** Have the mom switch to a prone position. Apply a firm and thorough massage for all back muscles, including vigorous massage to the rhomboids and trapezius and a focus on the low back muscles to loosen them up.

LOW BACK PAIN

Pain moves to the low back at the slightest provocation if the abdominal muscles are not strong. In my "training program" for pregnancy, a daily abdominal workout of sit-ups and crunches would be an insurance policy against a sore low back. But some women are already predisposed to this problem before pregnancy. If the mom has ever had a back strain, sprain, or trauma, then she should work hard to strengthen her abdominal muscles before any lower-back pain appears. This added stability for the low back will help with or often prevent any further problems. Massage lessens the tension in the back overall, and that will in itself help to prevent any buildup of pressure.

Low back pain may result from erector spinae muscles under habitual strain, chill, or trauma. It may result from sciatica or a disc problem or may involve the trunk side flexors that in pregnancy are working overtime. In pregnancy, any of these factors can help cause low back pain, which can sometimes radiate into the thorax, pelvis, and legs.

Some low back pain is caused by muscle spasms in the lumbar and gluteal area, especially in the latissimus dorsi muscles that go from the low back up the sides into the back of the armpits. Swimmers have well-developed latissimus dorsi, giving them a distinctive triangular shape to their back. Even swimmers can suffer from low back pain if they don't continue to swim through all semesters of their pregnancy and into postpartum.

The treatment of this type of back pain is an easy daily massage for the low back and hips. Your aim is to relax the contracted muscles to improve mobility and to strengthen the lumbar flexors, lateral flexors, and trunk rotators to provide stability. Focus on massaging adhesions at the attachments of the erector spinae, the iliac crests, the sacroiliac joints, and the gluteals. Then use additional kneading and effleurage to soothe pain and increase relaxation.

Since it may be too painful to massage the area most affected, focus your attention on the areas above and below the focus of pain. Apply heat and use effleurage and kneading strokes to encourage general stretching. Build the mom's tolerance for frictioning for any trigger points or adhesions at the border of the erector spinae, the iliac crests, the sacroiliac joints, and the gluteals. Don't be afraid to massage deeply to loosen adhesions, but let the mom be your guide about tolerable pressure.

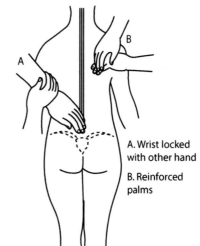

A. Wrist locked with other hand

B. Reinforced palms

Figure 3.38. Stretch the erector spinae with one or both of the two hand position variations.

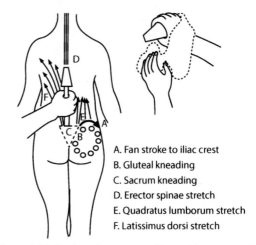

A. Fan stroke to iliac crest
B. Gluteal kneading
C. Sacrum kneading
D. Erector spinae stretch
E. Quadratus lumborum stretch
F. Latissimus dorsi stretch

Figure 3.39. Apply an ice massage. Dry melting water with a towel.

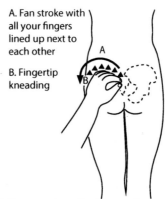

A. Fan stroke with all your fingers lined up next to each other

B. Fingertip kneading

Figure 3.40. Massage along the illiac crest.

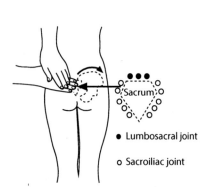

Figure 3.41. Reinforced or singlehanded fingertip kneading to the sacrum is useful for any kind of sacroiliac joint pain (usually felt in the low back and gluteals).

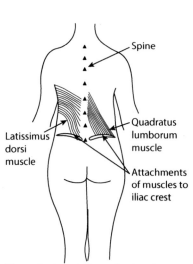

Figure 3.42. Latissimus dorsi and quadratus lumborum muscles.

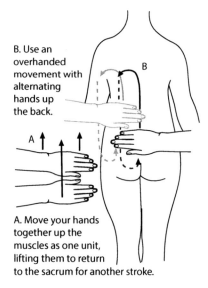

B. Use an overhanded movement with alternating hands up the back.

A. Move your hands together up the muscles as one unit, lifting them to return to the sacrum for another stroke.

Figure 3.43. Two options for palmar stretching to the latissimus dorsi and quadratus lumborum.

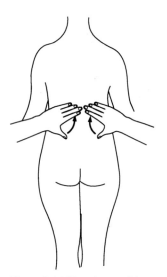

Figure 3.44. Thumb stretching to the quadratus lumborum. Move the thumbs toward the fingers, stretching the muscle underneath. Use both hands at the same time.

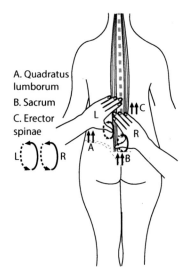

A. Quadratus lumborum
B. Sacrum
C. Erector spinae

Figure 3.45. Short stretching thumb stroke.

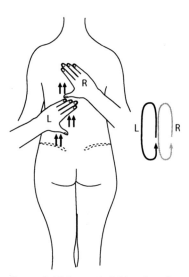

Figure 3.46. Long stretching thumb stroke to the quadratus lumborum and latissimus dorsi.

Lower Extremities

The lower extremities are especially important in the last two trimesters as they take the most strain with maternity weight gain. The symptoms of hip problems, sciatica, contracted iliotibial bands, knee problems, varicose veins, leg cramping, edema, and flat feet can all be treated with massage therapy. People with back problems often have additional symptoms of leg and foot cramping. They generally don't move as fast or as frequently as folks who are injury-free. With limited movement comes challenges to the circulation and the welcomed requirement for extra foot and toe massages.

Hip problems

Many women have problems with their hips before pregnancy. By the second and third trimesters, they may feel like *all* their problems are in their hips. The side-lying basic hip massage can be doubled, done on a daily or twice-daily basis, such as first thing in the morning and last thing at night. This will help the pregnant mom walk and sit more easily until she delivers.

Even women who have never had a hip problem before pregnancy may have hip problems during their last two trimesters due to a hypermobility in the pelvis caused by maternity hormone changes. A side-lying low back and leg massage will keep the tension from building up in the hip. See the massage treatment described in the second trimester, beginning on page 56.

Sciatica

Sciatica is described as a gnawing, tingling, or burning sensation in the low back, where the sciatic nerve exits from the spine, all along its path down to the lower leg. Some pregnant moms have sciatic pain before pregnancy due to an injury or lordosis. Others develop the condition during pregnancy, especially in the second and third trimesters as the pregnancy pulls the lordotic curve out of alignment, putting extra pressure on the sciatic nerve.

The best preventive measure is strong abdominal muscles. The stronger the abdominal muscles, the more stability in the pelvis and the less likely it is for the extra tilt caused by the baby's weight to cause problems. Strong abdominal muscles can resist the pulling of the baby's weight forward.

Massage to loosen up the hip area can help treat sciatica or even prevent it. I first met my patient Nadine postpartum when her sciatica, troublesome during pregnancy, became much worse after delivering her first child. With only a week's massages, the pain and discomfort began to disappear rapidly. I was able to leave her husband, Jeremy, with the ability to keep it permanently at bay for the rest of her nursing and recovery. This family treatment is ideal in postnatal sciatica in which the family can focus on both the mom's recovery as well as the baby's beginnings. When Nadine became pregnant a second time, she was worried her sciatica would flare up again. We worked on her hips and got the low back loosened up every week. Jeremy also gave a weekly massage and Sarah, Nadine's doula, provided a third weekly massage. So with three massages a week, she made it through the second trimester with ease, and so far, she is sciatica-free.

I massage the entire leg for all varieties of sciatica—small, large, persistent, intermittent, prenatal, and postnatal. The side-lying pregnancy-massage position is perfect to get the whole hip loosened up, which makes the sciatic nerve happier.

I often start on the unaffected leg to see what the real feel of my patient's leg is. I once started on the affected side and thought I had the treatment well covered, only to discover that the unaffected side was identical, although it had not exhibited any sciatica symptoms. My other rationale for starting my sciatica massage on the unaffected side is that the painful side is favored when walking, standing, or lying down. The unaffected side compensates for the painful side and does more than its share of the work of both legs.

SCIATICA MASSAGE (SIDE-LYING)

1. **Overhanded palmar kneading to the hip:** Warm the hip up thoroughly, usually with overhanded palmar kneading to the hip and gluteals.

2. **Fisted kneading to the hip:** Make fists and use them in the same motions over the hip for a deeper kneading sensation.

3. **Alternate thumb kneading to the iliotibial band:** Move on to alternate thumb kneading along the iliotibial band.

4. **Whole leg massage:** Do all the deep massage strokes (wringing, alternate thumb kneading, and thumb stretching) for the whole leg—including the low back and knees—as you would even without sciatica.

If the mom has a full-blown case of sciatica, then rest the leg and use ice frictioning with the pointed end of an ice popsicle on the low back lumbar area and the lumbosacral and sacroiliac joints (Figure 3.41). Use a facecloth or towel to catch the runoff of melting ice.

A person with sciatica deserves an overdose of massage and hydrotherapy. Use Epsom salt baths, ice massage, and alternating cold and hot water bottles to provide relief and stimulation.

Women with chronic sciatica may want to use a wheelchair toward the end of the pregnancy. The chair will help her keep up with the crowd for going to events or out for dinner. A pregnant woman with sciatica can receive a hip and low back massage right through her clothes while in a wheelchair or any other chair, even in the middle of a public event, so she can reestablish comfort and reduce pain without having to go home.

Most symptoms clear up once the baby is born, but sometimes they don't and became much worse after the delivery. In that case, you might want to get professional massage help.

Contracted iliotibial band

The iliotibial band is a band of fascia extending down the outside of the leg from the ilium (or pelvis) to the tibial attachment at the top of the outer side of the lower leg (Figure 2.15). This band is almost always tight, but a serious case of contracted iliotibial band is painful and restricts movement. In nonpregnant people this condition arises from too much or too little standing. Some people are more predisposed to this condition because they stand with their legs hyperextended, pushed back in an anterior bow-legged stance.

Your job is to keep this structure as supple as possible. This elasticity does not come easily. Sometimes I think that the extra elastin hormone in the pregnant body makes this structure change for the worse. The joints, being more elastic, can make the legs, low back, and hips hypermobile and loose. This will affect the naturally tight iliotibial band and give it more work to do to keep the legs stable.

The route of the band is usually very tender. Use effleurage, wringing, alternate thumb kneading, thumb wringing, and digital compression directly on the band. Repeat long effleurage strokes to "erase" the biting pain of the focused strokes so you can work into the area again.

STROKE MENU FOR A CONTRACTED ILIOTIBIAL BAND

1. **Effleurage:** to entire leg (3x).
2. **Reinforced palmar kneading to the hip.**
3. **Single-handed palmar kneading to the head of the femur.**
4. **Fingertip kneading to the attachments of the iliotibial band at the top of the thigh.**
5. **Alternate thumb kneading along the whole iliotibial band.** (Figure 3.47)

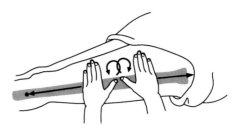

Figure 3.47. Alternate thumb kneading across the iliotibial band. Begin where the band originates in the tensor fascia lata and gluteals and run down to where it attaches to the lower leg below the knee.

6. **Wringing across the iliotibial band, including the quadriceps.**

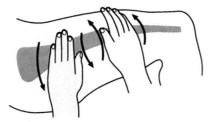

Figure 3.48. Wring across the iliotibial band, including the quadriceps. Use the wringing style shown here or an open handed C-shaped wringing.

7. **Deep palmar transverse frictions**: Use the thenar eminence (base of the thumb).

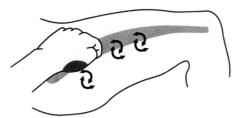

Figure 3.49. Tuck your thumb into your fist and friction across the iliotibial band using your thenar eminence.

8. **Long strokes**: Stroke along the length of the thigh going up to the hip, like a mini-effleurage, first with the thenar eminence (Figure 3.50a) and then with the thumbs (Figure 3.50b).

9. **Short strokes**: Move your thumbs forward and back in short strokes up the length of the thigh, always with pressure applied only toward the heart and just light contact on the way back. (Figure 3.50c)

10. **Transverse skin rolling**: Draw fingers toward stationary thumbs like a big pinch of the iliotibial band. (Figure 3.51)

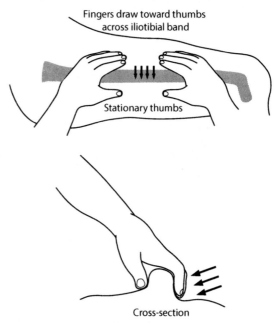

Fingers draw toward thumbs across iliotibial band

Stationary thumbs

Cross-section

Figure 3.51. Transverse skin rolling.

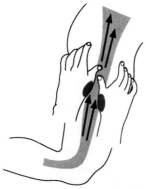

a. Long strokes with the heel of the hand. Use one hand or both at the same time.

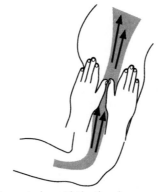

b. Long strokes with the thumbs.

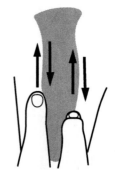

c. Short strokes with the thumbs.

Figure 3.50. Long and short strokes.

11. **Transverse stroke with the heel of the hand.** (Figure 3.52a)

12. **Transverse stroke with the thumbs:** Wring the tract slowly and deliberately. (Figure 3.52b)

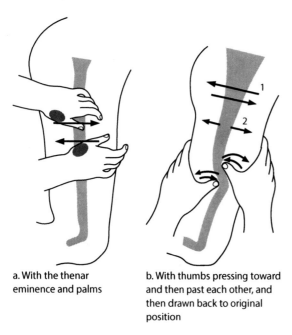

a. With the thenar eminence and palms

b. With thumbs pressing toward and then past each other, and then drawn back to original position

Figure 3.52. Stroke across iliotibial band.

13. **Reinforced palmar kneading.**

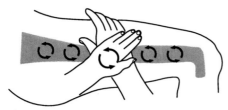

Figure 3.53. Reinforced palmar kneading.

14. **Wringing to the leg from the head of the femur to the toes.**

15. **Finish:** Effleurage and light reflex stroking.

Be sure to work the wringing and kneading strokes all the way down the iliotibial band to the attachment at the tibia past the knee joint. Linger at this lower attachment. This is where there is little elasticity because the iliotibial band likes to keep things inflexible and strong. You have to really work it as the weight of the baby increases and the legs are put under greater stress and strain until delivery. Women can also suffer a contracted iliotibial band postpartum due to carrying the baby.

At both attachments (hip and knee), but especially at and below the knee, use frictioning with ice or fingertips or a fisted knuckle. This back-and-forth movement helps break down adhesions. You can alternate kneading or wringing with frictioning to make the frictions more tolerable.

Knee problems

Bridging the top of the lower leg is the almighty knee, including the patella (kneecap). The knee is the largest joint in the body, carrying a fast-growing cargo soon to be delivered. But the joint is often not prepared for this instant jump in its job description. Swimming is excellent to exercise and strengthen this joint.

The most relieving stroke for any problems of the knee is wringing. I "slice" across the patellar tendon at the bottom of the kneecap. I also do a lot of frictioning around the perimeter of the kneecap, large oversized alternate thumb kneading around the outside edge of the kneecap, and fingertip kneading to the sides of the knee. If the woman cannot be comfortable on her side and can only lie face up, then do not forget to massage into the popliteal fossa (back-of-the-knee area) with some upward scooping strokes from the calf up into the back of the knee. See pages 40–41 for further discussion of massage for the knee.

Varicose veins

Varicose veins are lumpy, enlarged veins that usually appear in the legs. Spider veins, tiny blue or red veins on the surface of the skin, are a less severe form of this condition. Many women experience varicose veins for the first time during pregnancy, and those with varicose veins already may find they worsen, especially toward the end of the pregnancy when the growing baby slows the flow of blood returning to the heart from the legs. Varicose veins are challenged by gravity, weight gain, and standing occupations; they usually show signs of failure in the lower leg before the upper leg. Sometimes in the first trimester there will be small indications of this hereditary influence, with blue venules or tiny varicose veins appearing on the skin surface. This is usually more obvious in one leg than the other.

I avoid massaging varicose veins entirely and only use hydrotherapy to help relieve the congestion. Avoiding obvious varicosity showing itself through the skin is easy, but often there are things below the surface that are still to be skipped over. The mom will let you know where she has a sensitivity. I have a similar sensitivity in my lower legs that does not look at all obvious from the outside. Yet my legs react badly when someone massages my lower legs with any downward pressure, with my veins jumping up in protest. Those little gates only want to open up toward the heart. I am a walking advertisement for that principle of always keeping the pressure of all massage strokes up toward the heart.

For patients with varicose veins, use modified effleurage for starter strokes (skipping over areas with obvious varicosity) and then do alternate thumb kneading and wringing, always dancing over the areas where you see varicose or spider veins. Wringing is perfect for adapting to different sensitivities as you can change the pressure in a split second when the mom indicates a touchy or uncomfortable area. I always spend a lot of time on the feet of patients with varicose veins for a great relaxation response.

I had a patient years ago who was having her fifth baby. She had the worst set of varicose veins that I had ever seen. Her legs bothered her so much that I learned to use extensive light reflex stroking and light wringing, which provided her with immediate relief. My light, barely there strokes got her circulation going without causing more discomfort. We used a bucket of cold water and ice so I had cold hands for my light strokes.

Cold wet wraps on the legs can also relieve the congestion and pain. Those damaged, overextended vein walls react well to the constriction prompted by cold water temperatures. Cold leg baths and standing in cold streams are also excellent remedies for poor circulation in the lower legs. You can apply a cold leg wrap while you're massaging other parts of the body before and after your leg massage routine.

For a mom with varicose veins, be sure to elevate her legs during a full-body massage. Since you can't massage the varicose veins directly, a good place to focus your massage is the hips and upper legs, where no varicosity is present, but where you might be able to open up and improve the circulation.

COLD WRAPS FOR THE LEGS

Although the idea of wrapping your legs in cold, wet sheets might sound terrible, for pregnant women, especially those with varicose veins, a cold wrap on the legs is heavenly.

An absorbent flannel sheet works best. You may want to have two pieces of sheeting so you can wrap the legs individually. You will also need some plastic wrap, an extra blanket for insulation, some pillows, and possibly a hot water bottle.

1. Soak the sheet in a cold bath or container of ice water.
2. Warm up the legs with massage or by swimming or walking.
3. Wring out the sheet just until it isn't dripping. You want it to hold as much cold water as possible.
4. Working as quickly as you can, spread out the sheet so the mom can climb onto it and lie down, face up.
5. Quickly wrap the sheet around each leg separately and then cover the legs as tightly as possible with plastic wrap. You want to prevent air from getting to the cold wrap, which will heat it up. Wrap the legs right up to the upper thigh.
6. Elevate the legs on pillows and cover both legs with another blanket for insulation. You don't want the mom to heat up too fast.
7. If desired, keep the rest of the body warm with a hot water bottle under the neck. You can massage the rest of the body while the mom relaxes in her wrap.
8. When the wrap has heated up naturally (through the body's heat), you can repeat the cold wrap or just wash off the legs with witch hazel.

Leg cramping

Massage to alleviate leg cramps can be administered seated, face up, or face down. If the mom is prone to nocturnal leg cramping, elevate her legs with her in a supine position and use heating pads or hot water bottles to stave off cramping during this massage.

For my pregnant patients with leg cramps, I begin with the same techniques I use in sports massage for athletes with leg cramps. With the mom on her back, stretch the calf muscle (the gastrocnemius, a common location for leg cramping) by pulling her toes toward her head.

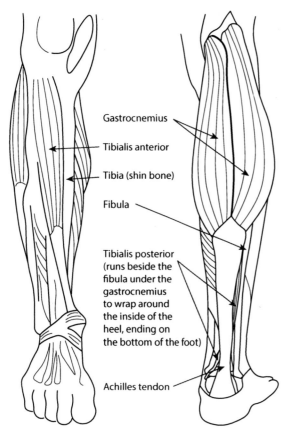

Figure 3.54. Lower leg anatomy. The gastrocnemius is a two-part muscle shaped like an elongated heart with a point at the Achilles heel attachment.

Alternating your hands, scoop up the calf from the Achilles tendon to the back of the knee, keeping the action and pressure sending blood to the heart for replenishment. It is like you are milking the muscle toward the heart.

Alternate these cup-shaped milking strokes with a more focused fingertip grooving into the middle of the fold of the calf muscle. Using the fingers of both hands, I put the points of my fingertips on the Achilles and "groove" into the calf muscle where it anatomically splits up the middle to the back of the knee. This divides the calf muscle in half, so I call this long stroke "splitting the gastrocnemius belly." On the backstroke, I put the calf muscle back together with a palmar kneading stroke across the lower leg. Repeat this movement at least three times, and more if wanted. Check after three, but the mom usually asks me to do this stroke forever as it affords her so much relief and feels so good.

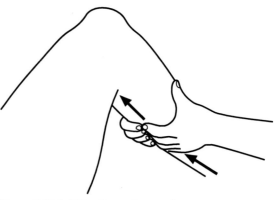

Figure 3.55. Splitting the gastrocnemius.

Once the tension is worked out of this hard-working muscle, follow it up with another massage favorite. Wrap your hands around the ankle like you are choking it. Your thumbs will be on the top and your fingers overlapping around the heel. Flex and point the foot at the ankle, providing a wonderful stretch to the calf muscle.

The cramping muscles of the lower leg don't stand a chance with this massage workover. Some people get leg cramping at night only. Elevating the legs for five or ten minutes at night before bed can help reduce swelling. If you're watching TV before bed, just lie on the floor with your legs resting on a chair.

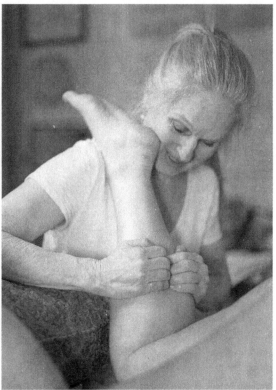

Figure 3.56. An alternative to splitting the gastrocnemius with the mom lying supine is to work with her lying prone. I like to bend the leg at the knee and lift the ankle up. I sit on the table or bed and lean into the angle of the leg while putting the ankle over my shoulder. With the mom on her stomach, you can also do some good alternate thumb kneading to the gastrocnemius. Wrap your hands around the calf as you work. Start at the popliteal fossa and work to the ankle and back again.

Most leg cramping, as in the low-grade achiness in the gums and teeth and other indications of calcium deficiency, are caused by the baby's development. The baby is parasitic and gets first dibs on nutrients in the mom's body. When I was pregnant, my teeth felt like they were going to fall out as Crystal thrived on my calcium! That feeling passed, but not without additional calcium in my diet. Check in with your midwife or healthcare provider if leg cramping is one of your symptoms in any trimester of your pregnancy. You may need a calcium supplement. Other preventive measures include keeping magnesium levels high and, of course, lots of massage!

Shin splints

Shin splints is a painful inflammation of the muscles, tendons, and other tissue along the tibia. They are a common complaint in pregnancy, especially among runners with a history of this injury. I always try to get my pregnant moms out of their running shoes and bikes and into the pool as early as possible in their pregnancy. It's great to keep their fitness level up, but pregnant women do better with a cross-training approach.

Locate the long tibialis anterior muscle next to the shin bone, to the outside (lateral) aspect of the tibia. This is where to do your alternate thumb kneading, up and down at least three or four times, followed by single-handed thumb kneading and thumb stretching. Follow the length of the tibialis anterior right down into the foot, where it attaches along the instep below the big toe. Be sure to be thorough as shin splints can be a very painful condition that will really slow down the mom.

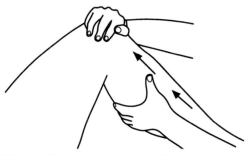

Figure 3.57. Supporting the leg with one hand, do some single-handed thumb stretching to the tibialis anterior.

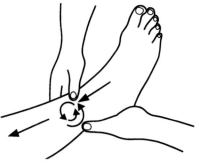

Figure 3.58. Cupping the heel with one hand, do some thumb stretching and thumb kneading to the tibialis anterior, with special attention to where it attaches to the tendon that connects the muscle to the inside of the foot.

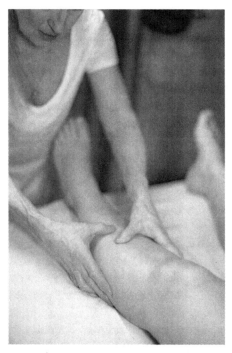
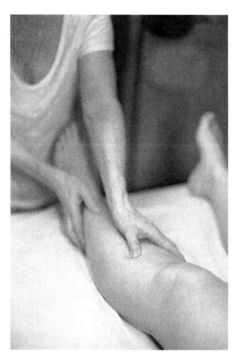

Figure 3.59. Overhanded thumb stretching is a series of short strokes about an inch or two long with a short straight stretching action. The thumbs move one at a time with one thumb picking up where the other one left off.

This is a good treatment for self-massage, at least while the mom is able to reach her shins! She can work up and down the tibialis anterior with her fingertips, like playing a keyboard.

With this condition, massage is important for the whole leg, not just the lower leg. Shin splints are difficult to get rid of once they arrive, so do all you can to prevent the condition. Make prevention a priority: with any hint of shin splints, get massage and hydrotherapy and head to the pool for an antigravity workout!

Flat feet

Prenatal flat feet is a weakening or falling of the transverse and longitudinal arches of the foot. Sometimes the condition occurs in the first trimester and then becomes worse as the weight of the woman's body forces the feet into further stretching and pain. You can start treating flat feet in the first trimester and continue beyond the end of the last trimester, into postpartum. In other words, this painful problem can go on for weeks and months.

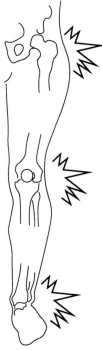

Figure 3.60. Pain caused by flat feet can be referred into the knee and hip.

The condition often has genetic sources. Anyone who has been more than forty pounds overweight may have experienced fallen arches. Pregnant women can have sore feet early on due to hormonal changes that oil their joints with extra elastin. This elastin is important for the mobility of the pelvis, but it does not restrict itself to just this area. The hormone is also very good at making the arches of the feet hypermobile, helping them spread and drop more easily. This can cause discomfort and often extreme pain, rendering some women unable to even walk. Prenatal swelling of the lower extremities can make this even more debilitating.

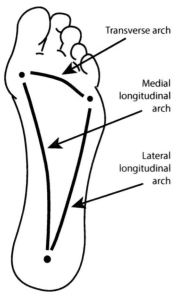

Figure 3.61. Arches of the foot.

The position of the mom for this massage can be seated, side-lying, or supine. Sore feet are treatable in the middle of the park, the airport, under the kitchen table, or at the bedside. This is an excellent TV-watching activity, especially around due dates!

The basic massage strokes of effleurage and wringing break up the surface tension of the swollen lower leg and start to establish a better flow of lymphatics and blood. I use the knee as the starting place for this routine and work around that area first to open up the circulation to the lower leg and foot.

The beginning of this massage is the same as the treatment of shin splints (see page 91). After splitting the gastrocnemius, focus your massage on the tibialis anterior, the muscle that runs down the front of the lower leg. This tiny highway of opportunity for relief is right next to the shin bone, the tibia. Because the tibialis anterior is the main muscle that helps hold up the proper angles of the foot, especially the longitudinal arch that runs along the instep, this massage is the best way to begin to relieve foot discomfort. You should be about one to two inches to the outer side of the ridge of the tibia. Follow that long muscle to its attachment at the inside edge of the top of the foot, crossing over at the level of the ankle. Use small, slow, firm strokes of alternate thumb kneading, fingertip kneading, and single-handed thumb kneading.

Move to open-handed wringing, alternating with long thumb stretching. This deep thumb stretching is the same stroke as the one done between the erector spinae and the spine while massaging the back. Use it now between the tibialis anterior and the ridge of the tibia. Move very slowly and be sure to be right on the tips of your thumbs for the greatest depth and accuracy.

After massaging the lower leg, continue on with the foot and ankles. A thorough foot massage begins with thumb kneading to the ankle bones and fingertip kneading to the attachments of the Achilles tendon to relieve any local discomfort.

Then you can begin some nitty-gritty strokes along the medial longitudinal arch that runs up the instep of the foot. First apply a mini-effleurage to the sole of the foot with your thumbs. Then move to thumb wringing across the medial longitudinal arch, alternating with thumb compression (just press each thumb in and hold for moment), alternate thumb kneading, and deep thumb stroking. With a firm touch, these strokes will give relief to this long arch. Encourage your mom to breathe deeply into each stroke.

The same sequence of strokes can also be done on the transverse arch at the base of the toes. This massage can be uncomfortable at first, but after about five minutes, most of this discomfort will subside.

FLAT FEET MASSAGE MENU

1. **Split the gastrocnemius**: Use both hands to split the gastrocnemius in an upward direction from the Achilles tendon to the back of the knee.

2. **Thumb stretching and thumb kneading to the tibialis anterior**: Single-handed.

3. **Thumb stretching to the tibialis posterior.**

4. **Kneading to the malleoli (ankle bones).** (Figures 3.62a and 3.62b)

5. **Thumb stretching to the top of the foot.** (Figure 3.62c)

6. **Thumb stretching to the medial longitudinal arch.** (Figure 3.62d)

7. **Static frictioning to the medial longitudinal arch.** (Figure 3.62e)

8. **Thumb stretching to the upper side of the foot**: Stretch in the groove between the long bones. (Figure 3.62f)

Figure 3.62. Massage treatments for flat feet.

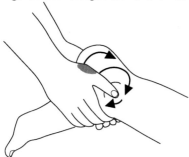

a. Kneading to the ankle bones (with heel of hand)

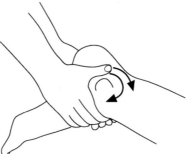

b. Kneading to the ankle bones (with thumbs)

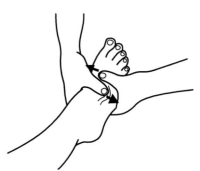

c. Dorsal thumb stretching

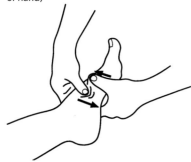

d. Medial thumb stretching

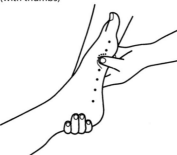

e. Frictions on the medial longitudinal arch

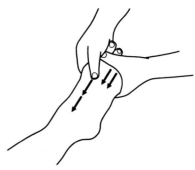

f. Thumb stretching

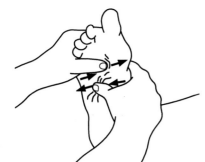

g. Thumb wringing

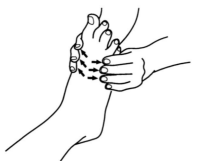

h. Transverse arch mobilization (dorsal view)

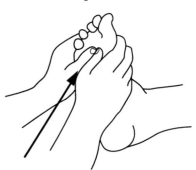

i. Transverse arch mobilization (plantar view)

9. **Thumb wringing to the sole of the foot.** (Figure 3.62g)

10. **Transverse arch mobilization:** with both hands, hold a foot at the base of the toes where they join the foot. Your thumbs will be on the bottom of the foot and your fingers on top. Working from toe joint to toe joint along the transverse arch, move one hand up and one hand down to mobilize each joint. (Figures 3.62h and 3.62i)

11. **Digital compression:** Alternate left and right thumb tips to apply pressure slowly and firmly all over the sole of the foot. Treat the sole of the foot like a series of trigger points, with the mom breathing into the steady pressure of each thumb. Digital compression is always the favorite stroke in this routine, but ask for lots of feedback to be sure your pressure is right.

12. **Frictioning to the medial longitudinal arch.** (Figure 3.62j)

13. **Frictioning to the joint at the base of the big toe.** (Figure 3.62k)

14. **Eversion/Inversion:** Twist the foot toward the inside and then the outside holding the foot with one hand and the ankle with the other hand. (Figures 3.62l and 3.62m)

15. **Transverse arch stretching:** Slide your hands from the ankle to the toes like you are squeezing the foot through your hands to make it longer. When you get to the base of the toes, bend the toes downward. Thumbs are on the top of the foot, fingers on the bottom. Then reverse your direction up to the ankle. (Figure 3.62n)

16. **Transverse arch mobilization with thumbs on top.** (Figure 3.62o)

Figure 3.62. Massage treatments for flat feet.

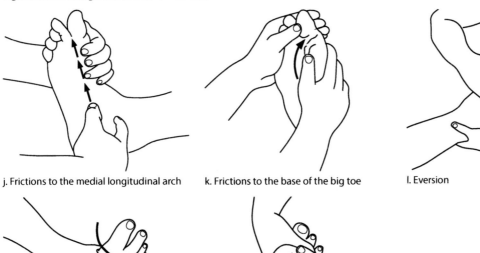

j. Frictions to the medial longitudinal arch   k. Frictions to the base of the big toe   l. Eversion

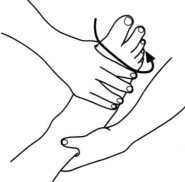

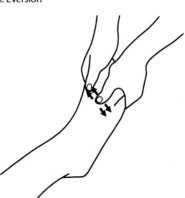

m. Inversion   n. Transverse arch stretching   o. Mobilizing the transverse arch thumbs on top

17. **Use your palm to flex the toes at the transverse arch.** (Figure 3.62p)
18. **Bend each toe up and down individually.** (Figure 3.62q)
19. **Alternate thumb kneading and wringing:** Wind down the massage with alternate thumb kneading to the entire foot (Figure 3.62r), a mini-effleurage up the leg to the knee, and wringing to the whole leg, especially the lower leg, right out to the toes to finish.
20. **Effleurage to the entire leg** (3x).
21. **Light reflex stroking to finish.**

Figure 3.62. Massage treatments for flat feet.

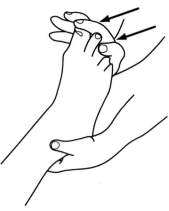

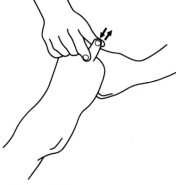

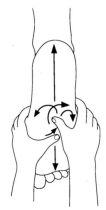

p. Flexion

q. Toe mobilization

r. Alternate thumb kneading to the sole of the foot

Flat feet can completely clear up in the first twenty-four hours postpartum, or they can stay with a mom forever. This isn't a problem if you married someone who can deliver a nightly foot rub in their sleep! Your kids will grow up with the right protocols.

There isn't a lot of good news for flat feet in the short, pressured time span of pregnancy. But the condition usually becomes more tolerable and treatable with not only hands-on help but also a lifestyle of swimming to keep those feet like healthy flippers. Footwear with style and healthy arch support combined is today both fashionable and affordable.

Running in the sand is good therapy for non-pregnant people, but running in the water is a better alternative during pregnancy. Pulling towels and washcloths around the floor with the toes will also help reform the transverse and longitudinal arches. Give that kitchen floor extra scrubbing to help those flattened arches perk up! Any gripping with the toes—gripping pencils, gripping sand, gripping fabric—are traditional exercises given by physiotherapists to help strengthen fallen transverse arches.

The more foot massage the better, combined with cold foot baths and any other cold applications of snow, ice, or freezing lake water.

Any of these maternity symptoms are a great opportunity for hands-on family bonding and intimacy. Everyone enjoys helping someone in need. Massaging someone's maternity problems helps both people—giver and receiver—feel good.

4

Massage for Labor and Delivery

This chapter outlines massages for early labor, active labor, pushing, and postdelivery.

Massage Positions During Labor

The key to labor massage is flexibility and adaptation. By this time, you will be used to the strokes and know what normally works best, but the mom might not be able to lie calm and relaxed in a face-up, face-down, or side-lying position. She may, in fact, be a bit of a moving target. In my classes, I try to get everyone prepared for three alternate massage positions (sitting, standing, and moving) that might be needed during labor. Learn how to get your body weight behind your hands so you can put enough pressure into your strokes in all different positions.

Sitting

When the mom is sitting, organize your posture to give the best pressure, usually a stride position with one foot ahead of the other. If you're standing at the side of the mom, you can brace your leg against one of the chair legs. This position stabilizes and saves your back.

If the mom is sitting on the edge of the bed, then you could be on the bed behind her in the shiatsu position, still at the side with one knee up and one knee down.

Standing

When the mom is standing in any position, put your weight onto your hands from your feet up. Don't rely upon strength in your arms and hands alone, as they will tire quickly. Lean or move forward to put your full body weight behind your hands. If you are not a big person, rock onto your front foot, lean forward, and distribute that hand pressure right down your arm.

If you are working from the side, put your back leg behind the person again in a stride posture. Never put your two feet together since you will not achieve the strength needed to massage from pregnancy to labor and delivery. You need to be always leaning into the massage from whatever position the pregnant person is in. You will be able to achieve more pressure and will preserve your back in the process.

Moving

For the moving target, you may need to hold on to the mom with one hand while you use the other to massage. For example, during a contraction, you might need to hold on to the mom's hip and use her as a counterbalance so you can exert pressure onto her lower back (sacrum). You support her so she won't have to work to resist your push.

Counterpressure Pain Management

The most important aspect of massage in labor and delivery is pain management during contractions. Although there are various methods of pain management during labor, I find that applying counterpressure on the low back is the most effective method for both pain control and increasing patient stamina. It is similar to the technique you learned for dealing with those sensitive trigger points around the body (page 59). The ideal massage for active labor integrates static counterpressure sacrum massage during contractions with full-body pregnancy massage between contractions. Your third trimester massages should practice all the techniques in this chapter.

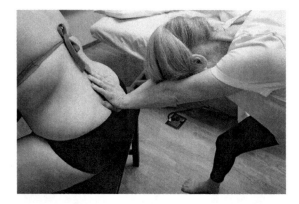

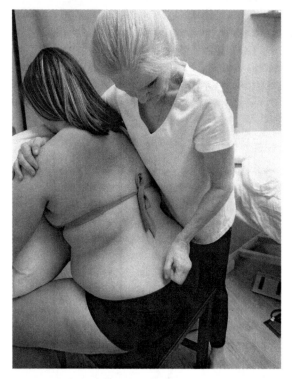

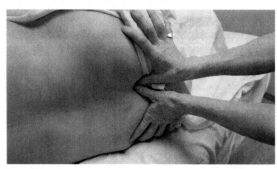

Figure 4.1. For counterpressure pain management, use your palms side by side, your fists, the heels of your hands, or your thumbs. I like reinforced palmar pressure directly on top of the sacrum.

For counterpressure pain management, press on one spot on the low back or gluteals from start to finish of the contraction. Try several locations until the mom tells you have the right place. This spot might change from contraction to contraction.

At the same time, talk to the mom, getting her to feel your hands and breathing into the pressure you're exerting. Use your voice to coach her: use her name and get her to breathe with you, slow and steady. Keep her focused on your voice and the sensation of your counterpressure. This technique helps the mom greet each contraction with a proactive approach. I find it is very strengthening for the woman in labor. Instead of feeling like she is under attack, she is going out to meet the force and use it to deliver the best results: a productive squeezing of her uterus to move her baby forward into the world.

The counterpressure of your hands, fists, or thumbs will give her choices in what she finds works best. Ask the laboring mom to give feedback about the proper placement: "Am I in the right place?" Ask this often as the baby moves farther down the birth canal and the pressure on the inside changes accordingly.

This hands-on teamwork is the essence of the labor and delivery massage and where I feel the most valuable in the work I do to help this process be the best it can be. The most essential technique of all maternity massage strokes, in my experience, is reinforced palmer pressure to counteract the acute discomfort of contractions. When I was in labor, suffering from persistent back pressure due to my posterior back labor, my husband kept his feet as counterpressure on my sacrum for hours. If your hands become tired, remember you have another pair of paws to apply.

Getting the Body Prepared for Serious Action

In the last couple of months, do your full-body massage, with or without the labor and delivery component, for at least an hour a day to develop the stamina you will need for the marathon of massaging required during labor.

This might seem like a huge undertaking, but it pales in comparison to the challenge that is the laboring woman's part of the bargain. The last phase of pregnancy is the most taxing on a woman's body. As the baby sinks down and presses against the door to the world, the woman feels pressure and may find her walking impaired. The baby's movement downward is a good sign of impending action, so pay extra attention to massaging the inner-thigh muscles from here on in.

I encourage pregnant women to "hatch" hot water bottles at any opportunity to sit. Sitting on heating devices keeps the floor of the pelvis soft, a good idea in preparation for childbirth.

You cannot do enough massage for the low back and legs in this time of waiting. If the extra weight of the breasts is causing headaches or tension in the shoulders, be sure the upper back and shoulders are included in your massage. Keep the mom massaged and ready for the event to start. This way she will be calmer and more flexible inside and outside for whatever lies ahead. So many of my patients have leaky breasts and painful shoulders in the last trimester's final days. All these "waiting for baby" signs are helped with your massages.

Massage around the due date is a great way to harness everyone's energy, anxiety, and excitement. During their visits, set mothers, best friends, and sisters to work giving daily or twice daily massage for the mother to be.

Massage for the Perineal Floor

There is a massage sequence that I never do but always suggest for couples to do. This is the massage to the pelvic floor, the perineal area "down there."

The perineal floor, that area between the vagina and anus, is a highly recommended massage homework assignment for the birthing teams in my workshops. The professional boundaries of massage therapy practice in Canada don't allow massage manipulation of this area, so this is a job for the mom's partner. Make this perineal floor massage part of the partner's massage routine for the last days of the pregnancy. Aim for about four or five times a week for the last four to six weeks

of the pregnancy. Studies have shown that women who do regular perineal massage before childbirth have lower incidents of episiotomy.[9]

The massage may feel uncomfortable at first, but any discomfort should subside after a couple massages.

Although most perineal massage described on the Internet consists of internal massaging, my approach is on the outside. The inside is taken care of at birth time, but the outside needs attention for the lead-up to labor and delivery.

Before beginning this massage, wrap hot water bottles or hot packs in towels and apply to the perineal area for about ten minutes. Then have the mom position herself in the "examination" posture with the knees bent and open. Support the mom's open knees with pillows so her legs can relax. The soles of her feet can be together if this is comfortable for her.

Be sure your fingernails are short and your hands are clean. I usually recommend using coconut or Vitamine E oil, but you can also use wheat-germ oil or another vegetable oil. Avoid petroleum-based oils since they can dry the skin.

1. **Thumb wringing**: Apply warm oil to your hands. Use the thumbs in a back-and-forth stretching movement. There should be enough room for three or four wringing levels, depending on how large or small the thumbs of the person massaging are. Work across and along the whole perineal area.

2. **Single-handed fingertip kneading**: This massage should move from general to specific strokes to achieve the stretch needed. Try a broader stroke first to accustom the area to your touch. (Hot water bottles ahead of time help here.) Use three fingertips together and then graduate to two fingers or even a single finger to increase the pressure. Be sure to massage slowly and firmly, working from the center of the perineal floor to the thigh, and then lift your fingertips up and start in the center again, working toward the opposite thigh. Stretch the skin out toward the thigh.

Support the leg that is leaning outward with your outside hand. Then, with a well-oiled inside hand, massage the attachments at the crease where the inner thigh attaches to the trunk of the body. Starting with three fingertips, knead slowly and firmly across the floor of the pelvis from one side to the center. After three fingers, you might try two fingers. With the pointer finger and the middle finger pressed together to act as one, apply small, slow, focused fingertip kneading to the perineal floor. Don't forget to check in about pressure frequently.

You may want to pause to apply warmth again before moving to the other side. Massage from that inner thigh to the center in the same way as you did for the first side.

I remember giving this perineal massage homework thirty years ago in one of my first pregnant partner massage classes, and a couple reported that the first time they tried this, the stretching they did stayed stretched. I will always remember the enthusiasm this class had for doing their perineal massages and how delicately they discussed their homework assignment. Checking in discreetly went like this:

> "How did the homework assignment go? How many of you did your assignment daily? How many three times a week? Anyone still hoping to do it? Did you see results in stretchability and softening? Benefits? Did anyone use hot water bottles before?"

At this point I ran a little quiz: "Remember, why is this a good idea? In what stages of labor is this applicable? What about after the baby is born?"

After the baby is born, the key word governing perineal massage is *ice*. I recommend ice packs and ice massage in postdelivery perineal massage, whether there is tearing or not, to calm the area and soothe any inflammation.

I advocate perineal massage as a daily routine, whether in partner massage or self-massage. Self-massage can be done in the daily Epsom salt bath. If doing a perineal massage as part of a self-massage routine, add in a leg and inner thigh massage as well.

The perineal massage is a great place for the home team to get hands-on. The massage is part of the pre-event training, but it can also be used during the actual delivery as the baby's head is presenting. This massage will help the baby deliver with a minimum of wear and tear.

Over the years I have watched many midwives massaging this area with the various goops, such as KY Jelly, that are bedside in the delivery room. The midwives go way beyond the stretching I encourage my couples to do. They will usually work the rim of the vaginal opening to make it as elastic as possible when the baby is crowning.

For couples, surgical gloves are not mandatory for this massage, but other people on the massage team should wear them to prevent any bacterial opportunity at the openings to the birth canal. This is the only time in maternity massage that I advocate the use of gloves.

Couples can never do too much perineal massage before labor begins. The stretching of the perineal floor can be done several times during the labor and delivery massages, not just once. During labor, I tuck in hot water bottles or hot packs covered in towels to the perineal area so there is

STAGES OF MASSAGE FOR THE PERINEAL AREA

1. Pre-event to soften and stretch the perineal floor ahead of labor (include in your full-body massage).
2. Labor massage for keeping the area open and ready.
3. Delivery massage around the opening, often performed by midwives. Some midwives use two to four fingers inside the rim of the vagina and manually stretch it round and round.
4. Postbirth perineal massage with ice stimulates the circulation and helps restore the tissues more quickly, plus it is reported to help relieve constipation, a common postdelivery complaint.
5. Remedial postpartum massage using contrasting applications of hot and cold packs to restore feeling to the area.

constant warmth. This warmth and the repeated applications of massage promote helpful elasticity.

The more this area is stretched and massaged, the better chance it has of responding to the enormous head coming its way!

Early Labor

Massage during the early stages of labor is good for building teamwork between the friends and family who will be involved in the labor and delivery. Onset of labor could be contractions once every hour for many hours. Full-body massage during this stage helps the laboring mom adjust gently to the force building inside her body. Use all the basic pregnancy massage techniques you learned in chapter 2. I advocate massaging whether you are in bed, walking, bathing, or doing yoga. Any way to keep the sleeping, resting, and relaxation happening is a great way to conserve the strength needed to do the hard work of pushing in the hours up the road.

Often laboring moms are still undecided about where they might deliver. I have been in a lot of labors that started at home and moved to the hospital when things did not progress after a good amount of time. In Nelson, the time to head to the hospital is when the contractions are one minute long and three minutes apart. Until that time, I massage along with the partner, as well as relatives and friends taking turns attending to the mom. Sometimes I orchestrate an army of volunteers, from siblings to the mother in law!

The highest number of people I ever had in the delivery room was ten, and somehow I managed to give them all something significant to do, massaging the mom without putting her into orbit. Keeping their hands busy was better than letting them all have conversations around the room, distracting the laboring mom from her focus. The partner in this case was very inclusive, which really helped.

A colony of people from near Creston were in one of my maternity massage classes at a local college. They were used to being together for births in their religious community. They had a banding-together vibe that was inspiring and gave me more insight into ways that I could coordinate large numbers so each person could have a proper place in the pain-management department.

It can be like a religious or spiritual experience conducting this dynamic through such a transforming time. It is easy to capitalize on the specialness of the event and control the energy in the room simply by giving people a hands-on job to do. Getting everyone going at the same speed and with the same strokes is an art.

Early-labor bathing massage

Many women like to spend their early labor in a tub, especially while still at home. Early labor is a great time to try out this water environment. There are lots of gaps between contractions to allow everyone to change positions from aquatic to non-aquatic without rushing. Sometimes the mom gets in the water and just stays there, especially if the labor speeds along so she can deliver in the tub. Other women move in and out of the water. Just follow the mom along and adapt your massage to wherever she is.

In early labor in a hospital, I spend most of my time leaning over the edge of the tub. As a professional, I am not allowed to be fully in the tub within the hospital setting. So I lean as far as I can over the edge of the tub to massage my patients in the water.

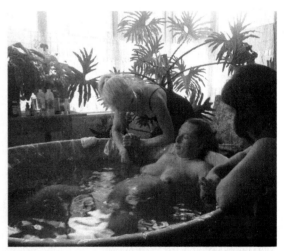

Figure 4.2. Holly chose to use the water to labor while the rest of her team massaged her from the edges of the tub.

But when in my patients' homes, I can work from either the outside of the tub or I can get into my bathing suit and massage in the pool, whatever is most appropriate for the situation (and the size of tub). Today, many home bathtubs are whirlpools that hold at least two people. Or sometimes luxurious birthing pools can be rented, some with room for four people. This is a big difference from the backyard wading pools we used forty years ago!

I encourage couples to try double bathing. At our hospital in Nelson, birthing partners can join moms in the tub. I always encourage dads and other partners packing for the hospital to make sure they put their bathing suits into the bag ready to go at the door so they can just put on their suit and dive in.

If you are massaging the mom from inside the tub, lean against the back and bottom of the tub to brace yourself to get the power you need to give counterpressure on the sacrum during contractions. I sometimes massage the laboring mom by squatting behind her while she is supported by another person or the side of the pool. This support ensures she doesn't float away from me as I push on her back in the water. Other times, I have to keep one hand on the mom to brace her while I push on her sacrum with my other hand.

When the contraction has subsided, use the warm water as your lubricant and keep massaging her legs and arms, baby, and back. The mom can move to sitting or reclining or side-lying, whatever she wants. Just adjust what you're doing to follow along. Sometimes I can be on one side of the tub massaging the mom while someone else is on the other side doing a tandem massage with me. Even if my massage partner has had no experience before, he or she can pick it up easily with side-by-side massaging together.

Social Media versus Massage

Today, early labor often becomes a conversation between people in different parts of the world. The advantages of Internet connection are miraculous, bringing into the room partners who would otherwise be isolated due to weather or work or any other

inability to be at the bedside. Grandparents-to-be in far-away places can be right at the fingertips of our couples in labor. Social media has also spread the popularity of labor massage, so more couples want to take advantage of its benefits.

However, I want those hands that are texting moment to moment to be massaging the mom instead. Today, the gaps between contractions are prime massage moments in danger of being eroded or invaded by technology. I was relieved when my daughter was in labor and her high-tech husband did not keep his family updated continuously about her progress. He was focused and centered on her needs. His hands stayed on her the whole time.

I am impressed with the way a lot of my families moderate their Internet addiction, even in a challenging situation like labor, where they can potentially feel helpless in the face of their partner's discomfort or fear. Many people turn to their phones at such a time out of habit, but I want everyone to focus on their laboring partner.

Early labor includes some of the last moments of the couple's life together as just the two of them. Within hours, their life as a couple will change forever. The massages in this phase of delivery have a staying power that provides the couple with lasting loving touch. These memories are locked into our bodies. We will always remember the last moments of tenderness, soft whispers into our ears of endearments and encouragement and gratitude. These are times for loving. If you must have a video of this event, arrange for someone else to take one.

Active Labor Massage

As the early labor shifts gear into longer-lasting contractions with shorter gaps in between, there is not the same sense of timelessness. Urgency starts to creep into the feeling of impending arrival, and we need to shift gears in our massaging. It is like coming around a corner and seeing a mountain in front of you. We have a momentum established; now we are on our second wind and heading to the finish line.

This is the last part of labor massage, and often the most short-lived part. We must use our hands and verbal coaching to help the mom breath into the sensation of the contractions, as they now get bitingly strong.

You will need to be more forceful with your directions, keeping the mom on a short tether. I try to be eye-to-eye and keep the mom with me all the way along the contraction. With the right touch and voice, I have been able to coach even the wildest of patients to loosen their grip. Often I am coming in on the labor at this stage of excitement. If the couple has not been hooked into each other, then getting the mom's focus and attention is like lassoing a creature on the loose!

You, too, can learn to use massage and words to direct her energy and collect her focus. Touch will cut through panic every time if you just give it time. With each contraction, the mom needs to breathe and focus on your hands on her low back. She can learn to tolerate the pain, and listen to your instruction to let go and let the sensation do its work. The discomfort is what we need; it is the baby's first, most critical massage.

The Importance of the Uterine Massage

In his book *Touching: The Human Significance of Skin*, Ashley Montagu describes the importance of the uterine massage during birth in stimulating the baby's nervous system. In all other mammals, which tend to birth more quickly and easily, the mother's tongue immediately reaches out to stimulate and massage her young; in humans, the tight squeezes given during the birth process fulfills this stimulating function. Montagu argues that the birth massage provided by uterine contractions is critical for the healthy physical and behavioral development of human infants. The more alternating pressure exerted upon the baby in utero, the more the baby's systems will be strengthened to start up on schedule when out of the uterus breathing air. This uterine massage works along the baby's body in exactly the way it needs. Though uncomfortable in the short run, it has big payoffs for the baby in the long run.

Tips for Active Labor Massage

The pressure the mother experiences sometimes warrants steady pressure on the back even in between contractions. When my daughter was posterior, the pressure was unbearable between contractions if someone didn't put pressure on my back continuously. With two feet on my back, my husband was able to keep me breathing and tolerating the pain for over twenty hours of unchanging pressure.

With my patients, I often use ice on the low back interspersed with massage and counterpressure. Wrap an ice pack, cold towel, frozen wet washcloth, or gel pack in a towel or sheet and apply it to the low back between contractions. Ensure the mom is warm before applying ice. You can wrap her in a warm blanket and put her socks on before applying the ice. When the pressure is overwhelming, I often apply counterpressure using an ice pack at the same time.

Active-labor massage is all about doing the massage like we are in a sports event. Be extremely flexible about when and how you do the labor massage. Just move along with the mom and massage what you can to help relieve her pain and prepare her for delivery.

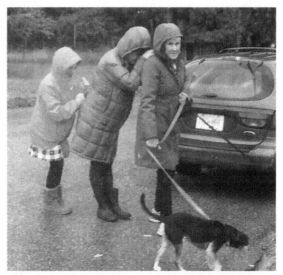

Figure 4.3. Flexibility is what active labor massage is all about. Here I am, pounding the laboring mom's back in the pouring rain as she leans on her mom. Yes, that's me at the back!

"Once my daughter Nadine's contractions started, Christine came to our house while we were all on alert and ready to go at a moment's notice. Christine's massages, especially on Nadine's lower back area, gave her a chance to get sleep for a few hours. The following day, the labor contractions continued, but not close enough together or intense enough to go to the hospital. At one point, Nadine wanted to go for a walk. So we took the dog and made our way up the hillside in Nelson. During contractions, Nadine leaned against a tree or parked car for support while Christine put her fists into Nadine's lower back. At several points, there wasn't anything around for support, so I became Nadine's wall as she held on to my shoulders while Christine worked on her back. I am sure anyone seeing us would have wondered what we were doing, but the right balance of massage, walking, and talking helped Nadine through her first stages of labor." —Wilma

Transition

When the contractions are one minute long and three minutes apart, we are heading into a transition on an undetermined timeline. We have to be ready, hands-on, for any change in momentum. We are eager to see our hardworking mom released from this test of endurance.

I have seen how massage helps restore and maintain the energy of the mom. Touch has a magical effect. Think of the Tour de France cycling race and how massage happens along the route in full view of the public, getting the athletes to peak in their performance.

The maternity finish line is just around the corner when the dilation reaches eight centimeters. Pushing time is quickly approaching, so you need to focus on keeping the mom from getting worn out. I am a big believer in naps between contractions at this point. If we had a total of the breaks between active labor contractions per hour (an accumulation of three-minute intervals) it would add up to over a half hour (thirty-six minutes, to be exact!) of resting and active rejuvenation for our mom to be! This is our massage reservoir. We accumulate over thirty-six minutes of hands-on massage interspersed with static counterpressure on the low back throughout that hour. That is a lot of ongoing recovery as the event proceeds.

Midwife Eileen Bell notes that although all the formal, textbook stages of labor are artificial mental constructs, they are still helpful as guides. I have often completely missed transition, that time of piggy-back contractions and no time in between, where the sensations of "needing to push" climax. Sometimes I will be massaging steadily through the labor and instantly there is the urge to push, and I rearrange myself to be ready for delivery. Sometimes, if the baby is already sitting low when labor begins, there is a building urge to push throughout the labor, whether it be short or long.

Pressure on the cervix

As the baby's head drops, pressure on the mother's tissues becomes increasingly intense from her hips down to her toes. Although this pressure is needed because it helps thin the cervix and dilate the tissues to permit the baby to travel out of the mom's body, it is nonetheless very uncomfortable for the mother. You can ease the feeling of congestion in the lower extremities by really concentrating your massage on the mom's hips. Releasing the tension in the hips allows the entire birthing area to open up. This massage is usually done with the mom in a reclining posture, which will lighten the pressure of the baby's head on the cervix.

You can never do too much massage to the hip area at this point. If the woman is lying or sitting on her back face up, you can lever your hands underneath her hip to work the area. If she's on her hands and knees or squatting, you can still apply all your variety of hip massage movements between contractions. Massage for the perineal floor may also help.

Once the baby is past the cervix, it's a whole different ball game. Now your job is to ensure the muscles do not spasm. Focus on opening the thighs and keeping the mom's legs wide open. Get more aggressive and really work the inner thighs as the baby's head crowns.

Inner thighs

The inner thigh muscles have a tendency to reflexively tighten up against the contractions. Ideally, get two people involved in loosening this tension, one massaging each leg. Face your massage partner and massage each leg in tandem, with the same rhythm and strokes. This will help build a sense of team bonding. Start by massaging the inner thighs with wringing, wrapping right around to the hamstrings in the back of the leg.

Follow the wringing by single-handed alternate thumb kneading and fingertip kneading. Hold the bent leg at the outside of the knee with your outside hand, and with your inside hand knead with your thumb and fingertips. I use wringing every few minutes to smooth out the more focused strokes and make the area not feel so "pokey!"

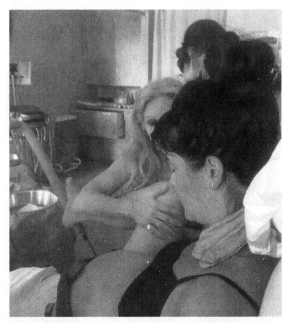

Figure 4.4. Nadine's inner thighs and entire leg were massaged when her feet were in stirrups during contractions.

Avoiding cramping

Cramping in the lower extremities, especially the calves, is a common symptom of great exertion. Massage the legs firmly and actively to get the blood moving. Using this sports-massage strategy, I am able to get the birthing mom through the active, transitional, and pushing stages without spasms in the legs.

The birthing mother is often plagued with cramping all the way through the active labor and into transition, and then it disappears. But sometimes the opposite is true, where the birthing mom has no cramping and then the spasms start up after the delivery, as they do when athletes are on the massage table after the race and their legs spasm due to lack of oxygen. Keep your hands on the birthing mom and you will work out uncomfortable sensations before they build to a spasm.

As the baby's head works its way to around the pubic bone, the pressure suddenly shifts for the laboring mother. Spasms can appear in places that were not a problem up until now. For example, the gluteals (rear end) can go into spasm, as can the inner thigh adductors. These cramps are uncomfortable but short-lived, and can be treated with quick hands-on massages. Use all massage strokes, including just gripping and squeezing the spasming muscle until it lets go. Very firm wringing and kneading is critical for getting the mom through this difficult phase of delivery. Be sure the mom is breathing deeply; as in sports, many spasms occur because the body is not getting enough oxygen during a long workout.

Delivery

Pushing requires a change in strategy and focus for your massage. Your goal is to help the mom get the best results in pushing. You want long, productive pushes with major squeezing of that baby, and to accomplish this, you need a mom with energy. Pushing is a feat of second wind and endurance.

For pushing, you want to harness every ounce of her energy and focus it into pulling her legs back and wide. I usually hold a leg on one side and have a nurse, midwife, or birthing team member hold the other leg. Hold the heel of the foot up in the air with the bent leg leaning as far out and back toward the mother as possible. Usually I am supporting the leg with my entire body. This position really helps the bearing down to work. When everyone is hands-on working together, it is a wonderful team feeling, and has been from the first time I delivered through to my most recent delivery last week.

Then, in between contractions, drop the legs and start massaging again from thigh to toes. Ideally the massage team has more than one set of hands on the job at this point. Intensely focused on this intrepid aspect of the delivery massage, we keep up this pace of whipping the massages onto and around the resting woman, massaging until the next push. Work the inner thigh, iliotibial band, quadriceps, and hamstrings, all attachments around the knee and the lower leg, and especially the gastrocnemius (calf muscle), where cramping muscle spasms most often occur. Use the routine massage stroke classics:

- **Lots of firm, rapid effleurage**: Remember, pressure toward the heart, light on the way back.
- **Enthusiastic wringing**: Work on one leg while someone else does the same massage on the other leg. Wrap the wringing all the way around the leg and under, working the hamstrings and the quads at the same time.
- **Alternate thumb kneading**: Work the whole thigh, with focus on the inner thigh.

Move rapidly from massage to pushing, with quick gear shifting (usually double clutching!) to hold that leg and keep the knees as far apart as possible during pushing.

During pauses in the delivery pushing, coach the mom to let everything go and drop down, conserving her strength. Vigorously massage her shoulders, arms, and legs, and get someone else to put hands on her sacrum, which helps with the overwhelming pressure in the low back. This isn't easy if the person is in a face-up position, but you can still slide your hands under her back and lever your hand (or both hands) up into her sacrum.

Stay there, with steady pressure, during contractions, then slide your hands back out and continue massaging between contractions.

Massage Team Positioning

Although I have attended kneeling deliveries where the mom is on her hands and knees, I have the most experience in face-up deliveries with the mom holding her legs behind the knees and the rest of us supporting her ankles, feet up in the air. The dad or other birthing partner is at the head of the operation, head-to-head, heart-to-heart with the mom. He has the job of lots of verbal coaching. Or, if there are just two of us with the mom in the labor and delivery, dad may be on the other leg. But these days that is rare, and more common is the team consisting of the mom, mother in law, best friend, doula or midwife, the hospital maternity nurses, and, of course, the father to be or other partner. Again, in this end stage of labor and delivery, it is really important to keep the crowd hands-on with the birthing mom.

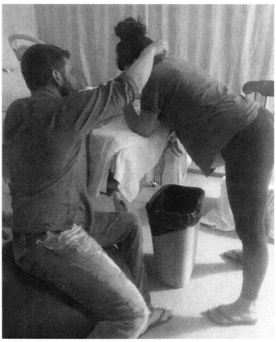

Figure 4.5. Hands-on dad, head-to-head.

The best massage team would have the dad cheek-to-cheek or nose-to-nose with the birthing mom, a shoulder massager, two leg massagers, and our midwife/care provider. That totals five hands-on helpers.

With four massagers, two can be on the legs, one with counterpressure on the sacrum, and one eye-to-eye coaching the mom. With three hands-on massagers, put one on each leg and one with counterpressure on the sacrum.

A TEAM EFFORT WITH LOTS OF COACHING

My son in law was steady with his coaching of my daughter throughout her labor, counting her along while I massaged as soon as the push extinguished itself. During Crystal's pregnancy, I wasn't sure how Joel and I would do as far as teamwork went, as Joel is the most independent person I have ever encountered. From the first practice contractions, however, Joel seemed comfortable with my hands-on presence and we were a great team.

All the massage before and after the epidural had Joel and I massaging Crystal through her nausea. We massaged her back when she turned on her side to have her epidural administered. I was lucky to have Joel working with me. He's a strong-handed, hands-on type of person with an intuitive understanding of Crystal's aches and pains. She was able to withstand both of us working on her at the nth hour of the proceedings, at least partly because she was used to lots of massage.

She had suffered with extreme, often debilitating menstrual cramps throughout her adolescence, and my techniques for those pains were the same as for these pains, in the same area and with the same type of talking: "Take it easy, Crystal. Just let everything drop down. Let your shoulders drop all the way down to your fingertips. Just let your whole back drop onto the bed and feel the warmth of the blankets wrapped around you. Feel my hands working on you and let the relaxation sink in and sink down. Keep breathing deep and let it all go." This part of pushing was the part that I had practiced over the years with Crystal's cramps: "Just take a deep breath and breathe into my hands."

I always have nurses and other helpers massaging the legs and sometimes I am the one nose-to-nose with the mom while the dad is watching the baby come into view. After the baby is out, the massage team keeps working the legs and gets ready for the postpartum delivery of the placenta.

The leg holding, the counterpressure on the sacrum, the pause that refreshes between pushes: all these duties are the exciting teamwork of the delivery. The big finale is in reach. All medical staff are on board and the room is humming with activity.

Do not be intimidated by the invasion of staff and equipment in the final moments. Keep massaging the birthing mom. She needs the steady focus of your hands now more than she needed anything you might have done in all the laboring massages. Now is the time to get her over the finish line.

The Last Push

Now we are pushing. This is where the touch of the farmer is needed. I learned delivery massage in the barnyard long before I thought I would be a massage professional. I've seen more than one farmer massage up the birth canal of a Holstein cow with an entire arm inside the cow, turning the calf so it would come out the right way. I have now seen midwives and doctors perform similar massage feats. Common to both is the need to stretch that opening in the final stages to allow the birth to take place.

Working the opening

When the baby's head is crowning and obviously ready to pop through, it is important to work the lower edge of the vagina to stretch the tissues to accommodate the baby's delivery and ensure a smooth glide out. Every time the pushing sensation subsides, the midwife or physician will tuck fingers inside the rim to reinforce the stretch. If they can't get an edge of the finger inside the rim, they'll just keep stroking and stretching along the surface of the edge with their fingertips.

Now we have the most perfect pausing where the mom learns to hold off on the seemingly uncontrolled urge to push, and the midwife or physician can ease the baby's head gently out beyond the thinning lip of the vagina without tearing it. Thinning this out is a last-minute massage accomplishment done with the finest of touches.

The stretching massage along the vaginal edge can never be overdone if it is done the right way. This edge is tough tissue with heavy muscle. Its normal sphincter action has to be turned off for the baby to slide out. Although the therapeutic clipping and nipping of an episiotomy has helped many a stuck delivery to release its hold, ideally a massage can ease the baby through the opening without requiring any stitches.

The midwife from whom I learned the most about this stage of massage for delivery always places a supportive hand on the perineal floor to prevent tearing while massaging around and around the rim of the vagina with the other hand that is coated with medical goop or coconut oil. This massage, along with warmth applied with hot towels or water bottles, is the best way to stretch the circle wider as the baby descends.

I am convinced that this massage has saved many women from tearing or from needing an episiotomy. Even with the tightest of vaginas, there is an opportunity to coax the tissue to stretch. Midwife Eileen Bell says, "I think you have to be in touch with the tissues of each woman, letting your fingertips tell you her story. As the baby's head appears, the delicate dance of responding in the moment will still be at your fingertips. Your hands will tell the story."

After the placenta: knead, knead, knead!

Placentas are like babies: they deliver themselves. We don't need to worry or do anything special to help them along.

Some countries have superstitions about the placenta. When I was teaching midwives in a countryside village, the birthing position was traditionally squatting with the women fully clothed and people surrounding her for physical and emotional support. A tight band was cinched around her above the baby and pulled tight to prevent her from swallowing the placenta. Although this traditional practice was based in folklore, I felt like I was doing something sacrilegious to tell them any different.

How long had that myth been keeping birthing moms from being able to take deep breaths during their labor and delivery? Loosening the cinch and teaching the gathered midwives breathing with massage and pressure focused on the sacrum is still one of my most treasured teaching experiences. I loved the way the midwives were keenly interested in learning new ways of helping the pain of childbirth.

Counterpressure on the low back combined with the opportunity for the laboring woman to lie back and have her legs off the ground was a new birthing alternative for them. However, part of what they were doing with the cinching, which kept pressure on the uterus after the baby and placenta were delivered, was brilliant. That therapeutic pressure was and still is perfect for helping the uterus contract quickly. An intense uterine massage will help with muscle fatigue and will encourage the uterus to tighten down and not leave itself open to bleeding.

The most vigorous uterine massage I ever saw was at one of my first births. I saw a midwife knead the mother's abdomen with extraordinary force as the mother's blood pressure plummeted. The massage caused the uterus to clamp down, stopping the bleeding, and the mom's blood pressure normalized. Since then I have witnessed more of these therapeutic uterine massages.

All the midwives and medical professionals I have helped with these uterine massages have taught me different techniques, but all do the massage with forceful strokes. Some use a slow, deep kneading action to get the uterus down into a firm ball, while other midwives quickly alternate between scooping into the abdomen and fisted kneading strokes.

Sudden Changes

When a C-section is called for, your role changes to a more passive position. You need to be able to quickly change tracks to support the mom in what may be a physically and emotionally trying time.

I am often invited into the C-section with or without the birthing partner or other members of the team. I love keeping the mom calm and relaxed while watching all the medical intervention. I am often the mom's eyes and give her a running narrative while I massage her shoulders and neck.

The first time I was asked to stay with a birthing mom through her C-section, I had a fractured jaw due to a dental problem, and my experience of the C-section had an ethereal quality to it totally separate from the birthing experience. Whenever I had my hands on my patient, the pain in my face and jaw disappeared. When I took my hands off her shoulders to do something like adjust the curtain or shift my posture, the pain was instantly back. That phenomenon of being connected in this way has forever blessed me with insight into the power of touch.

In this somewhat passive role, usually sitting at the head of the mom, sometimes behind a curtain that completely blocks the operating area and attending physicians, I still am able to do massages for the mom's head, neck, and shoulders to help calm and relax her, especially if she has had a lot of pushing and is fatigued or has sore arms from holding her legs. This upper body massage can be very rejuvenating and relaxing.

With my patient Ashley's C-section, her mother and I were able to massage Ashley's legs to help her involuntary shaking subside. We felt lucky to have an important job to do while the rest of the family gathered in the hallway outside the operating room.

Whether your baby delivery is *au naturel* on dry land in the hospital or home, a water birth, or a C-section, the adaptation of massage to all these birthing scenarios is seamless.

Post-Birth Massage for Moms and Babies

The arrival of the baby signals the end of the labor and delivery massage and the beginning of the postpartum massage. Even with a C-section, the baby is usually quickly placed in the mother's arms so skin-to-skin bonding can take place, even while surgery protocols continue. The completion of every effortful event, be it a wedding, sports event, or study marathon, has the same feeling in the aftermath: overwhelming relief.

In postpartum, our focus is the mother's recovery, the start of breastfeeding, and family bonding. We want to speed up recovery from the aftereffects of the fast, slow, or textbook-normal deliveries. Sometimes I can start massaging the mom's head, neck, and shoulders while she holds the baby in the operating room. Other times I start my postpartum massage while the newborn is nursing in the recovery room. I just adapt to whatever position and circumstances works for all of us.

This massage is a celebration and reward. Get the mom's favorite special oils; get cleansing equipment, such as a bucket of hot water, handmade soaps, and lovely washcloths. Whether you are in the hospital or at home, the mom's first massage in the baby's life is very special. Have all these supplies ready to go for the first hour after the birth. Massage all the extremities thoroughly in this postevent sports massage for faster recovery. It's time for teamwork again in a softer and quieter manner while the baby sleeps.

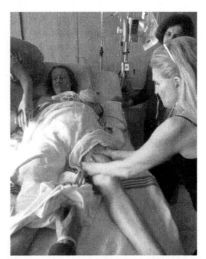

Figure 4.6. Mom can cuddle the baby while you give a postevent sports massage to ensure her speedy recovery. Don't be concerned about any medical activities around you—just get in there to massage the mom's legs and back.

Postpartum Massage

Postpartum massage is designed to be restorative. The exertion of labor and delivery, be it short or long in duration, is intensely physical. Massage helps restores circulation, which helps body tissues rejuvenate more quickly. This chapter outlines ideas and techniques to encourage quick recovery and greater stamina for the challenges of postpartum: the new work of breastfeeding, coping with lack of sleep, or healing from delivery trauma. The combination of massage and hydrotherapy is especially effective for speeding the recovery from any type of special delivery: prolonged, breech, C-section (planned or unplanned), or instant arrivals!

Beyond physical recovery, the power of touch helps moms who suffer from postpartum depression. For some women after delivery, the hormonal roller coaster levels out smoothly, but other women find it a challenging time. Responses to hormonal swings can range from serious depression to a milder twenty-four-hour crying jag. We can massage for all postpartum symptoms: emotional, physical, and spiritual.

The First Twenty-Four Hours

The mom

Even moms who had straightforward, relatively easy births need a massage, just like any other athlete at the end of an event. If possible, provide two massages in the first twenty-four hours: one immediately following the birth in the recovery room, and the second later on the first night.

The new mom's physical challenges range from massageable muscle strains to the aftermath of difficult deliveries, including stitches and hemorrhoids that can cause the new mom to be unsteady on her feet. Moms who have had epidurals may now have a heightened sensitivity in the low back. They may feel heaviness in the legs or a "funny" feeling in the feet. Putting the mom's feet back under her is an immediate, practical goal. She needs to be able to hold the baby with confidence and walk with balance. You don't have to give an elaborate massage: even twenty minutes makes a difference.

For these first postbirth massages, give a general overall massage to the entire body without digging into any specific area. The tissues are usually fatigued and the mom may appreciate a relaxing massage with large, superficial strokes and a soak in an Epsom salt bath. In the first twenty-four hours, I encourage the mom to lie face down (with good pillow support) to press on the uterus.

You want to be sure to get at the mom's back, even briefly. You may be able to deliver this massage with the mom in a side-lying position, or the mom may be face up. In that case, you will need to work your hands under her body, levering your fingers up into the back muscles. If you had a massage partner during labor, get that person to help you with a tandem back massage down both sides of the spine.

When my daughter delivered with the help of an epidural, she quickly recovered steadiness on her feet and stamina due to massages immediately after her delivery. We massaged her back while the baby was being weighed and measured, which encouraged the symptoms of her epidural to make a speedy exit. This was in the first few minutes and hours after my granddaughter was born.

Our massage helped her to tell how the epidural was wearing off. Each time we massaged her back, she could feel our hands more; she was starting to thaw out and every massage over the next few hours gave her feedback about how her process was unfolding. We were able to massage her to sleep.

Sometimes the epidural does not wear off quickly and seems to gently take its time to fade. Massage of the legs, hips, and low back are important to do in this first couple of hours, even if the mom's sensation has not fully returned. The effect of revitalizing these places will be felt when the feeling does return. I worked on Crystal's legs many times that first day with a focus on her hips while she breastfed in a side-lying position.

Crystal says the foot massages she received stand out in her memories of her massage marathon. Her feet had been swollen for much of her last trimester, and they seemed to swell even more during the labor. This is a mom who was massaged frequently, both before the labor began, and then by both her partner and me throughout the fourteen-hour labor. You could say that she was the most over-massaged mom in history, but still her legs swelled up!

A breast massage in the first few hours after delivery is also important to ease up surface tension in the breasts and help colostrum production. This is especially appreciated if the patient has had a lot of breast activity in the past few weeks. See chapter 6 for details on breast massage.

Those without any medical intervention during labor and delivery are still flooded with postpartum hormones. The massages we deliver in these first hours postpartum are memorable if only due to the heightened sensitivity of the new mom's skin. Hormones help create an even stronger sensation of touch.

Birth partners are usually not as available for massaging as they were predelivery. I therefore rely on mothers, mothers in law, girlfriends, and family for this first stage of postpartum massage. This is why I like to teach an entire neighborhood of friends so that the postpartum massages never stop.

FEELINGS OF LOSS

New moms sometimes feel a physical sensation of loss after giving birth. The body can take time to adjust to the absence of that comforting, moving, live presence inside her. Having a new baby is definitely a positive loss and a great gain, but it still takes time to adjust to the new emptiness.

People often get in touch with their bodies by having a massage. I sometimes don't realize how tight I am until someone puts his or her hands on me. I hear this every day from my patients. They come in for one problem, but then they realize that the problem stems from another location simply by the information they gain when I touch places they cannot get to themselves.

In this same way, massage helps the new mom assimilate the dramatic changes in her body and feel comforted in the emptiness and often aloneness in that "once full, now vacant" center of her body. That little "buddy" has flown the coop, often leaving a feeling of physical loss behind.

Use warmth, preferably with a bit of weight, for the abdomen to comfort that hollow space. I like the hydrocollator packs that are conveniently located in the birthing wing of our hospital. They are heavy and the perfect baby size and weight. A hot water bottle or beanbag also provides good, comforting pressure—better than lightweight heating pads.

FIRST NIGHT MASSAGE

You can usually give the mom a full massage after the crowd clears and the relatives go home. If they know she is getting her massage within the first couple of hours after delivery, that seems to work well for helping the clan vanish.

The second postpartum massage is for the mom's full body. Massage all the extremities and the back, especially the low back. Use all the rejuvenating strokes, from long effleurages to specific wringing, palmar kneading (reinforced and single handed), thumb kneading (alternate and single handed), and reinforced fingertip kneading to ease out tension and encourage restoration. Remember to concentrate on the shoulders and hips when massaging the extremities to open up the circulation to the arms or legs.

Massage the mom's back with her side-lying or face down. The mom has probably not been on her abdomen for months and this massage is often the first time for her to lie face down. Position pillows and rolled towels to support her breasts and let the abdomen press against the bed. The pressure of the weight of her body against the shrinking uterus is therapeutic. It is similar to the old-fashioned practice of putting the big family bible on the tummy to compress the uterus.

After giving birth, many moms have increased levels of appreciation for pressure. What the mom might have felt as a firm massage before labor might now, with her new hormonal levels, feel like a normal treatment she can easily tolerate.

Importance of couples' massage

Ideally, new parents would be massaging each other the first night after delivery, but usually the new baby becomes the focus of both parents. If the daily massages from the dad were to continue for the next month as they were in the month before delivery, tactility would be in balance. But I have seen many moms suffer from the withdrawal of their partner's touch.

The couple massaged each other through the pregnancy training period. They successfully finished the marathon of touch through labor and delivery, and now they need a postevent massage that is so important to restore their reserves and help them establish their new relationship, which just added another tiny person. The abrupt change emotionally, physically, and spiritually is mediated by touch and the medium of massage.

The first night postdelivery is a great time for the new dad to give the postpartum mom a full-body massage or mini-massages. This is also a time for the dad to get a massage for himself. He can get his feet or shoulders massaged while holding the baby.

I had a birthing couple that were so good with their massages for each other that the aftermath of their baby delivery was filled with massages. They massaged each other and then the baby and then they started all over again. Postpartum massage in the postbirth glow of the new family is a special time. A loving touch has the power to heal the wear and tear of the last twenty-four hours and ease everyone into the new reality of being a family instead of just a couple.

When the baby is sleeping, that is the perfect time to reestablish the skin-on-skin comfort and nourishment that is so needed to re-bond. I encourage new parents to take the time every day in that first week to touch each other with foot massages; head, neck, and shoulder massages; and full-body massages. They take the energy from each other and revitalize their relationship, generating a deeper level of intimacy. As with babies, skin-to-skin contact is good for couples.

Most birth partners are highly receptive to hands-on involvement in this recovery phase. They enjoy the opportunity to show their appreciation for the mom's hard labor and delivery work by lending a helping massage hand. Birthing partners are often really good at going between the baby and the mom with massage enthusiasm. I enjoy teaching these partners everything I can to equip them as the best Canadian maternity caregivers.

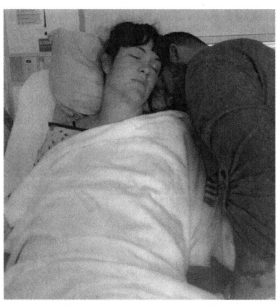

Figure 5.1. Whether they are in the hospital or at home, the couple will ideally curl up with each other and add the touch of massage to that overall body contact, comfort, and appreciation.

The baby

The first twenty-four hours is also a time for the baby's first massages. At the busy northern British Columbia center where my daughter gave birth, skin-to-skin contact was the focus. Posters promoting this early bonding contact are posted everywhere in the birthing wing. The birthing team is also proactive about being hands-on for a healthy, strong start to baby's life. Paige was rubbed constantly while being weighed and measured. Crystal's breasts were encouraged to be active, with lots of good latching on from Paige. This early suckling was part of the hospital's baby-arrival protocol.

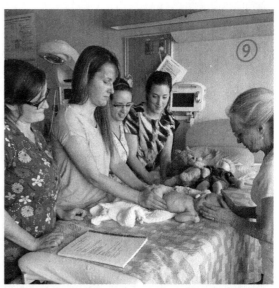

Figure 5.3. Teaching baby massage to the maternity staff at the Fort St. John Birthing Centre. Nurses in maternity care can teach baby massage to new parents before they leave the hospital to equip them with the best home skills possible.

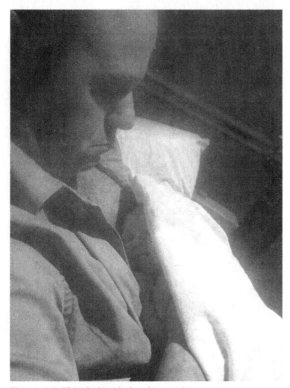

Figure 5.2. This dad took the skin-to-skin contact promotion very seriously and wore a button-down shirt to the delivery to ensure he could provide the baby with this early connection.

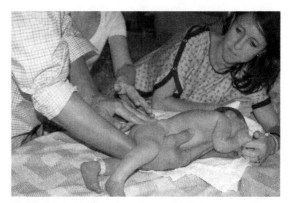

Figure 5.4. I will often show the couple baby massage basics on the bed beside the mom. Sometimes the dad and I or a brother or sister will be the ones to do the first baby massage while the mom looks on. The mom's breastfeeding can create an instant bond with baby, so it's great to have something dads can offer baby on an equal status with mom.

I encourage pregnant couples to attend baby-massage classes when they are still pregnant. I have babies arrive at the end of my pregnant partners classes so the pregnant couples can learn the basics of baby massage. These new parents share their babies with the pregnant couples in a great community-building gesture.

The support and camaraderie are instant. Look on YouTube for "Mountain Baby Massage" and you will see a dad teaching another new dad his

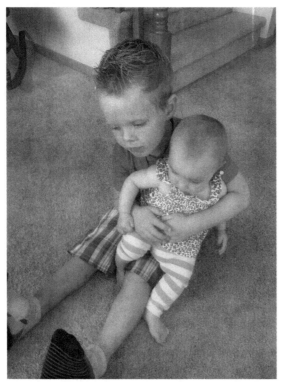

Figure 5.5. Siblings can learn massage to help them ease into their new role as big brother or sister.

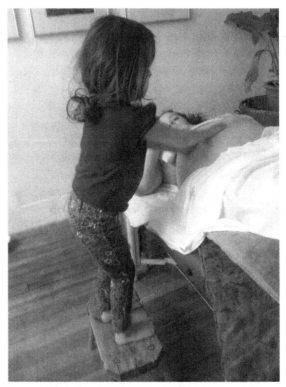

Figure 5.6. Having the whole family hands-on ensures the new baby is a welcome, not threatening, arrival. Even young children can have an important role in massage before and after the baby arrives.

variations on my instructions. For me this was wonderful. The connection between the dads through the baby massage was endearing, like a special boys' club.

Through baby massage, the newborn becomes bonded with the family. Both parents can work together on their newborn. Massaged kids grow up with a sense of natural touch that is calming, soothing, nourishing, and bonding. This attachment through touch is an ancient art perfected by our couples today.

The team

Once mom and baby are taken care of, I turn my attention to the team of massage volunteers who just completed their marathon of support. It is great for everyone to experience restoration through the power of touch. Form a circle and rub each other's shoulders, be they mothers-in-law or best friends, husbands, or maternity nurses. Everyone deserves the power of appreciation that comes through the fingertips.

I place the dad in front of the nursing mom and work on his shoulders as the last massage I do in the birthing room before I retire to massage the staff at the nursing station on my way home.

All the postpartum massages that Crystal got in the hospital were sought after by the staff, with teasing comments about sharing her mother with the rest of them. Many encouraged Crystal to move over so they could get the same treatment. Little did they know that my professional follow-up in the first twenty-four hours or immediately postpartum is to massage the whole team.

The reason for this important protocol is not as obvious as it appears. When the mother sees everyone getting massaged, she is immediately able to relax herself. She knows her team is well looked after, and her new mothering instincts can now stay focused on the baby.

While families spend important quiet private time together after the delivery, I do as many head, neck, and shoulder massages as I can for the team at the nursing station. In Nelson, this team includes doulas, midwives, labor and delivery nurses, student nurses, floor clerks, nursing coordinators, doctors, pediatricians, and obstetricians. The whole team, including the surgical team, are on the massage list for head, neck, and shoulders. Every time I massage the staff in the nursing station after a birth, I let the family know that the nurses just received their tactile box of chocolates on behalf of the happy family.

This is the power of touch. The staff usually can't think of anything more fitting for a thank you, and through this book hopefully you will take this postpartum time, this first foray into domestic family massaging, to the outer reaches of the birthing team.

The First Week

One of the surprises in the first week of recovery is the postbirth hormonal storm. This can range from feelings of depression to daily crying. In this first week of being a new mom, the physical and emotional changes and challenges seem to peak. Again, massage is your ally!

Thirty-five years after giving birth to my daughter, I remember that by three o'clock, my stitches usually throbbed, my feet hurt, and I would cry at everything. By five o'clock I was completely out of gas. I was "lucky" that my hemorrhoids gave me a great excuse to lie down anytime, anywhere. My husband recognized this pattern after a couple of days at home and gave me a pillow and blanket, making me lie down on the couch to sleep at 4:30 on the dot. Those naps were memorable. They were so restorative that I could feel the difference just a half-hour sleep could do for my outlook on life (my new life) and my physical stamina. Without

Willie's insistence on my nap, I would not have been able to focus on myself and the new baby.

This first week at home with the new baby is a special time. I don't see some of my couples during this week because they carefully separate themselves from the outside world and concentrate on this precious time of new beginnings. Often the dads only have that first week off work, and they want to do everything they can for their new family. The self-sufficiency of the couples harkens back to our Canadian roots of only a hundred years ago, where the men were more hands on because the midwife might not arrive in time for the birth.

I encourage couples to prepare ahead for this cocooning time. Practice different scenarios for postpartum massage while you are still in the pregnancy massage phase. In my workshops, we go over the massage and hydrotherapy combinations for breast care and then for perineal care if stitches, tearing, or hemorrhoids are factors. I recommend practicing the cold-towel breast wrap and postnatal breast massage in the last month of the last trimester. Details of these are found in chapter 6, which is devoted to breast massage exclusively.

Hydrotherapy

In the postbirth phase, if the mom has stitches or any length of episiotomy, then she will want to have applications of ice and cold compresses for the entire outer pelvic floor. When I had extensive stitches from my daughter's delivery, I found that Epsom salt baths were a godsend. I also took that little hat with holes that sat on top of the toilet seat seriously. I was able to soak myself a few times a day.

Ice massage stimulates the healing tissues and speeds recovery. I recommend ice popsicles to work around the incision site, always moving the pressure of touch toward the incision. Take care not to tear any healing incisions—your massage has the goal of increasing circulation to the area, not to deeply work the tissues. The same massage methods for perineal massage can be used postpartum by the couple as long as they are careful to always massage with pressure toward any incision site, not away from it.

HOME REMEDIES

In rural areas, gardens were once full of herbal remedies for all stages of pregnancy and delivery. People around the world have also traditionally used water in therapeutic ways, whether from soaking in medicinal hot springs or using full-body wraps of different kinds to stimulate the body's natural desire to "right" itself, restore balance, and heal.

I was very lucky to live with Russian Canadians in the Kootenays, who taught me the uses of our local plants and their application for every ache and pain, including cures for maternity concerns. The following home remedies are the ones I recommend:

- **For stitches or tears**: an Epsom salt bath (3x daily).
- **To sleep better**: deep-breathing exercises with massage and exercise in the fresh air for twenty minutes (3x daily).
- **For better circulation in the feet**: Use the Kneipp method of cold water contrast foot bathing (see page 31).
- **Other circulation enhancers**: cold breast wraps (page 127); abdominal wet sheet wraps; frozen perineal pads soaked with witch hazel.
- **For the baby's digestion**: Avoid any gas-producing foods such as cabbage, broccoli, and chickpeas.
- **To prepare the nipples for breastfeeding**: I recommend that pregnant women toughen their nipples using facecloths, toothbrushes, loofas, and anything else that has texture. This old-fashioned preventative measure has produced positive results with many of my patients.

Old-fashioned linseed compresses were still being used for postpartum abdominal treatments at Women's College Hospital in Toronto when I started working there in 1980. I loved learning about the traditional methods of postpartum care such as hot towels, hot water bottles, and frozen witch hazel pads for perineal healing. All such methods, whether ancient or contemporary, try to achieve one thing. They are applied directly onto the abdomen or perineal area, restoring circulation to the area of rehabilitative focus.

FIRST WEEK ABDOMINAL MASSAGE MENU

1. **Heat**: Apply hot water bottles to the abdomen and a heating pad to the back.
2. **Effleurage**: Up and down the abdomen.
3. **C-shaped scooping**.
4. **Reinforced fingertip kneading**: To the digestive system, especially the lower colon and corners, where things can slow down.
5. **Wringing**: Across the abdomen.
6. **Lifting**: At three levels (diaphragmatic, waistline, sacrum). Work very, very slowly (3x at each level).
7. **Vibrations**: To the entire colon and extra care to the descending colon where things can back up (constipation).
8. **Overhanded palmar kneading**.
9. **Light reflex stroking**.

If the mom is constipated, add in some leg pumping, or walking or squatting can help. Side-lying hip massage can also activate the pelvis and abdomen.

Now, one hundred years later, I thank that great Canadian, Alexander Graham Bell, for helping me. The phone is a great tool for staying connected if the postpartum couple is on retreat. I often use FaceTime or Skype to answer patients' requests for advice or help. With Skype, I can massage a pregnant or postpartum mom at my end of the connection while my patients follow my instruction to massage in their own home across the country. Technology is especially good for postpartum massage, which can be done every day the first week.

First week massage routine

First week massages should be daily at whatever time works well for the parents. Usually a full-body massage with a focus on the abdomen and breasts is what is needed most.

ABDOMINAL MASSAGE

I suggest you do an abdominal massage with all the same strokes you used in the first trimester pregnancy massages, including the constipation treatment strokes. This will encourage the digestive system's peristaltic action, good for helping with hemorrhoids or constipation. This abdominal massage is effective in moving bowels that might be slow, sedated by pain medications, or constipated from the trauma of birth.

Moms with C-section stitches on the outside have further stitching on the inside. For their post-surgical postpartum recovery, use gentle, superficial massage to the abdomen around the incision site and bandaging. Be careful to make the direction of your strokes toward the incision line, which is usually horizontal at the pubic bone. Underneath that outside incision, the layers of incision run the other way. If there is a C-section involved, keep everything gentle in the first week of massage to the abdominal area.

BREAST MASSAGE

The breasts go through huge changes this week, so daily breast massage is not enough. This is the week to massage the breasts a couple of times a day. I recommend that moms do a mini massage before and after breastfeeding. Do all the basic breast massage strokes (scooping, kneading around breast attachments), but for only a short time. Do the strokes for five minutes or less per breast or even for both.

As life with the baby is very much governed by the breasts in this first week, I encourage people other than the mom to learn the mini massages. The dad or other parent is also a good candidate for this lovely ritual, which allows him an important skill to help with milk flow. The breasts might not give our mom any trouble, but I like a twice-daily full breast massage and the minis before and after breastfeeding as a preventative measure against engorgement. When the breasts are hot and bursting even after breastfeeding, try holding a freezer pack and then performing the massage with icy hands.

This contrast can also be achieved by dipping hands into a bucket or bowl of ice cubes and cold water. The contrast between hot and cold is extremely helpful in getting the engorged blood in and out of the milk ducts. Chapter 6 has more detail on breast care.

MASSAGE FOR NEW ACHES AND PAINS

Some women's symptoms of sciatica do not appear until after the birth. The same is true with contracted iliotibial bands, knee problems, and flat feet.

Many women's bodies adapt to all the physical changes of growing and carrying the baby during pregnancy without comment. After the birth, there is a sudden shift as the load the woman was carrying is no longer an issue, but the body is still in its prenatal pattern of adaptation. The body does not always jump to change; some adjust rather slowly to the freedom of movement they have now received with the baby's delivery. The muscles do not always know what to do.

I have had patients who are much worse after the delivery, with symptoms down their arms and legs that seemed manageable during their pregnancy right to last push. Massage treatments of the symptoms of pregnancy are also helpful now in this next phase. Ask the mom what she's feeling and add in new routines, if necessary, to address new aches and pains.

Get on top of any uncomfortable symptoms and to address postsurgical issues with a combination of modern and traditional methods. Be friends with cold-water applications in all forms, including ice massage, compresses, or ice packs for the private parts.

Hormone regulation

As every mother knows, hormones change quite dramatically during pregnancy and after birth. The hormone changes play an important role in ensuring the mother's body is a good host for the growing baby. But in addition to the physical effects, the shifting hormones can make some women feel extra sensitive and emotional. Massage can provide physical and emotional reassurance for the pregnant and new mom.

SUNLIGHT CURE

An old-fashioned (but effective) treatment of speedy recovery of the perineal floor is the sunlight cure. I remember a story of a famous actress who was badly injured in a back-alley abortion. She not only used hydrotherapy to speed up her recovery, but also ultraviolet radiation. She exposed her private parts to the sunlight to "tan" her wounds and promote healing.

That story always stayed with me, and I have promoted this technique of wound recovery to many palliative patients suffering from pressure sores. Putting whatever part of you into the sun will help the wound site heal faster, provide an antibacterial boost, and help the wound dry up quicker.

My friend Joni, who is now eighty-six years old, had eight births in her lifetime. I will let Joni tell her story in her own words:

> We did not have a hospital near Grahamdale, Manitoba, in those days, and although I wanted to have my babies at home, my husband, a farmer, said that he birthed pigs, horses, and cows, and had no intention of birthing humans. He made sure I was in Winnipeg at my parents' house at least two weeks before my due dates.
>
> This was sixty years ago when you were in the hospital for ten days, and as both of my first births happened rather quickly, I needed stitches for both. I well remember the blanket-covered cage they put over my upraised knees every morning and evening for at least an hour. My naked butt was raised on a pillow under the cage, and a sunlamp shone down on my exposed body. When I asked the nurse what it was for, she reassured me that it was sunlight that we could not get any other way under the circumstances, and it helped to heal the stitches and to keep that critical area healthy.
>
> I really did not have anything to compare it with, but when I sat under that light I did not feel as much pain as during the hours in between. This went on for nine of the ten days before I was released from the hospital with my new baby.
>
> When we were ready to have our third child, we then had a nine-bed hospital newly built in Ashern, Manitoba, and the hospitalization time after childbirth had been cut back to four days. When Art was born, he was over nine pounds and I again had many stitches. They did not use the sunlamp at the tiny local hospital, but I remembered about the lamp when I got home, and since we raised baby chicks in the spring, we had our own lamp.
>
> I got my husband to put a hook in the ceiling over our bed and hang the lamp from there, and after I got the first two down for the night, I would do my own sun treatment in the open room with the door shut. I think it really helped the stitches heal and helped me to be more comfortable. We had just got electricity into our house that spring, so I was glad I could use something I learned from my previous experience in Winnipeg. I definitely feel that it helped the healing process. If nothing else, it forced me to have an hour in the evening to just rest, because running a farm with two runabouts and a new baby really wore me dry.

Joni's story is one of ingenuity and resilience. The massages that are now given to Joni in her eighty-sixth year are part of her lifestyle, with the goal of staying healthy and supportive for the next generation of babies. The massages for her in her senior years are the same massage techniques that would have been useful for her pregnancies and postpartum stages: leg massage, lower-back massage, and a focus on the hips.

"Fourth Trimester" Postpartum Massage

All these first-week massage practices carry forward into the rest of the first month and the entire fourth trimester. In the first month, the mom's mother, mother in law, and all her visiting aunties and close friends are the perfect daily massagers! Areas of focus include the following:

- Head, neck, and shoulder massage to ease breastfeeding tension
- Arms, for breastfeeding challenges and carrying the newborn
- Upper back, especially between the shoulder blades in the rhomboids, which can be painful due to breastfeeding and wearing the baby with slings and carriers
- Low back to address any continued issues from the pregnancy or the labor and delivery
- Legs, especially if the mom has sciatica, which can prevent her from being able to move around

Use your pregnancy-massage routine and massage the whole body slowly. This full-body massage adapts to include the new focus for breastfeeding and remedial recovery from any labor and delivery traumas. For prenatal women who experienced swelling in the lower extremities, massage in the fourth trimester will relieve that swelling, this time for good!

Breast massage in this fourth trimester helps to prevent mastitis and engorgement, and helps all types of milk production. Remember also that your touch can also help calm hormonal swings.

As we transition in this book to a focus on breasts and then baby massage, I want to give you a schedule that will take you to the completion of this postpartum maternity massage cycle.

Ramp down schedule for massage in the fourth trimester

- First week: daily
- First month: three times per week
- Second month: twice a week

- Third month on: once a week for the next nine months or as long as breastfeeding continues

Loving the unlovable

Postpartum touch can be, well, touchy. Postpartum moms may be grateful for your loving tactile care, but they may also be momentarily unable to express those positive feelings to you. You may, in fact, be forced to love the momentarily unlovable.

I once attended to a fellow massage therapist when she had her baby. This woman was normally someone who appreciated my massages, but in the week after her birth, she was edgy and detached from her partner, so much so that I thought maybe their relationship was in trouble. In addition, she had an almost obsessive focus on the baby, not allowing anyone else to touch him. This angry, edgy, overly protective behavior was completely out of character for my friend.

The whole time I massaged her postpartum, I felt like I was unwanted or an intruder. I persisted, however, and saw the gift of touch work its magic. The massage helped her relax and unwind. In short time her anxiety disappeared.

I remember feeling so emotionally fragile after delivering my daughter and then again after I had an ectopic pregnancy. I had lined up massage from two friends each time, but my friends, for perfectly valid reasons, had to cancel. I was devastated when they canceled, instead of a more normal reaction of mere disappointment. I looked fine on the outside, but inside I needed a massage to help me cope.

So remember, she may look normal on the outside, but on the inside a postpartum mom can be suffering. Assume the need and start with the solution: "Where can I massage you?" instead of "Do you want a massage?" "How can we arrange you to be most comfortable?" instead of "Do you feel comfortable?"

Then, once you have your hands on her, you can assess the situation with all that tactile information at your fingertips. I always get a box of facial tissue and keep it close in case it's needed. I encourage the mom to tell me her concerns (I try not to use the word *worry*, but that's what I'm after). When there is a high need, the massage is memorable for both people. I always operate best in high-need situations as it seems to bring out the best in me.

A recent high-need massage was my young neighbor giving up her baby for adoption. Two of us, her neighbors, supported her through those weeks leading up to the birth and for the month after the birth with the most hands-on massage help I have ever done in all these years of maternity massage. Her need was high and nothing else could have healed her hurting heart better than our loving touch. It was postpartum massage at its finest.

"I think my pregnancy was fairly healthy overall, because even though I didn't have a proper partner to support me, I was fortunate to have Christine and Sarah Yarwood help me through with the massages. Without the massages, I would not have had any physical contact. I think the massages were good for the baby as well, especially because of how the homeostasis of the mother affects the child.

Christine also led the adoptive couple and me through a massage for my daughter Kamala after she was born, and that was truly a beautiful experience. It was so important to help the adoptive parents get comfortable making physical contact with Kamala.

Finally, the postpartum massage helped me through the very intense emotions of being without the baby I had just given birth to. It was definitely one of the hardest times in my life, but I was able to stay positive and help heal my body with daily massages for my first thirty days." —Erin

---

Massage for Depression or Loss

Postnatal depression is unnerving when you have all the joy in the world to celebrate with your new baby, and yet you somehow feel sad. Long, hot Epsom salt baths can help speed up the hormonal adjustments. Every time I had a long soak and sweat, I felt relieved, not only of my aches and pains, but also of my delicate emotional state. I didn't feel so thin-skinned. It was as though the bathing did a massage on the inside of me.

The power of loving touch through massage has a miraculous effect on physical symptoms as well as emotional ones. The body cannot hold out against caring touch; massage helps soften even the hardest of heartbreaks. New moms need that touch more than ever before as they adjust physically and emotionally to their new position in the world. Even with an easy delivery and delightful baby, the mom may still feel momentarily lost or disconnected as her body and psyche catch up to the changes. This is an important time for spouses, family, and friends to forge a hands-on connection with the new mother.

In case of a tragedy, massage becomes even more important. After my ectopic pregnancy, I was not able to do anything but sit with a heavy heart. I eventually sought help from a counsellor and grief recovery group, but in the immediate aftermath, the hot water bottles on my tummy were comforting in all departments: physical, emotional, and spiritual. I had four hot water bottles: one between my breasts, one on my abdomen, one between my thighs, and one at my feet. The warmth of these objects helped substitute for the warmth of being held when no one was around to hold me through that rough time. I was very lucky to have a hands-on husband who massaged my back from the time I started losing the baby through my operation, my recovery, and the grieving depression that followed. Before my husband went to work, he tucked me in with hot water bottles. This was a lovely signature and a tactile extension to his loving touch.

The body experiences a surge of excitement to greet a new baby and then a drop off a hormonal cliff when loss occurs. That kind of hormonal roller coaster is very different from natural live births with real babies to cuddle. After losing my ectopic pregnancy, I had no baby and was crushed.

The miracle of touch was not administered by my fellow professionals but rather by my male carpenter friend, Leon. I remember his healing touch to this day. He was able to help me let go of that place inside me that was full of pain and suffering and lightened my burden with his wonderful massage on the floor of our master bedroom. Of all the massages that I have experienced, that massage was the most powerful. The love I needed was provided with Leon's healing touch.

Today, I use a combination of warmth and massage with all my loss patients. I help the person plan a professional visit a couple of times the first week, and then a team of loving friends to keep the healing happening. Your loving touch through massage can help work the grieving along its course and prevents emotional paralysis. Often the tendency is to leave people suffering loss to themselves—this is often what they demand as it is the body's natural instinct to suffer alone and keep away from lively energy or laughter. But the answer is the opposite. People need to make contact and be held. Pain can be soothed by contact, and pain can pass into the essence of the loss without the agony attached. Animals do a great job as therapists for loss because they can sleep right up against us and soothe the heart of a suffering mother, father, brother, sister, grandmother, or friend. Wrapping my arms around my rotund little dog helped me make it through many painful nights following my own loss.

Often there will be locations in the body that hold more pain than other locations. This is the nature of pain withheld. It is not a bad thing that the pain of loss is held tightly protected on the inside. It is natural to store up the pain. The person might not be in an emotionally safe place to be able to release such keening.

But once the touching rapport has been established, the woman can thaw out emotionally and keep the feelings flowing out of her. The power of touch can be soft as a caress or traditional as the kneading of muscles, both having the potential to ease the tension of suffering. The comfort of love and affection from a spouse, family, and friends adds to the healing power of touch in the face of disappointment or tragedy.

Palliative pediatric massage

Sadly, there is a place for palliative pediatric massage. It is a mother's greatest fear—losing her baby, yet even in this trauma, massage can play a role. I will let my patient Ellen tell her story about the last days in the life of her son Sebastian in her own words.

"I'm happy to share my experiences and hope that they will enrich your book and help others. I think that you asked me once before, and I was not ready—but now I am.

I didn't do much massage with the boys when they were babies. I remember that you came over and taught us how to massage Isaac when he was a newborn—and I remember going to the Chinese medicine school where you demonstrated on Ronan. Those were awesome experiences, but I didn't make massage a big part of our lives. (Or maybe I did and don't remember! Life with newborns is intense—especially when there are one or two preschoolers running around too!)

My memories of the time with Sebastian are very vivid, though.

In earlier admissions (when he was not on a ventilator), I could hold and carry him, and that's what I did most of every day. After a painful procedure—and there were many (blood draws, lumbar punctures, skin biopsies, suctionings, and so many more), I would scoop him up, dive into the rocking chair, and nurse and cuddle him.

At home, most of every day was spent holding and rocking him. That was as soothing to me as it was to him. Being held and rocked relaxed him and seemed to ease his pain.

The last hospital admission was very different. His last ten days were in the ICU at BC Children's Hospital. He was eighteen months old. We were in a private room, and he was intubated (on a ventilator). He had numerous other attachments too: an NG tube, oxygen prongs, an SAT monitor, and more. Because of the ventilator, I could not pick him up. There were few free areas on his body that I could even touch. He was old enough and aware enough to be very, very unhappy. He did not want to be soothed in the old ways. If I tried to sing his familiar songs, or show him photos of his brothers, or tell him familiar stories, he became very distressed. It seemed that he was saying, "Those things are for home. I don't want anything to remind me of home while I am here in this horrible place." I had to be creative to find ways to soothe him. I remember that I played with his toes a lot. I pretended that they were piano keys, and I "played" classical pieces on his toes.

I asked to be able to hold him. Some nurses were not comfortable with that, but some nurses would let me. It was a big production. I sat in a chair close beside his bed, and it took a couple of nurses and an RT to unhook all of his machines, transfer him to me, and hook them all back up. As soon as we were settled, he would relax. You could tell by looking at the numbers on his monitors that he was relaxed and comfortable. We could stay there for a couple of hours.

One day we had a young, creative male nurse. When I asked to hold Sebastian, he gave the matter some thought. Then he called for helpers, and he picked up Sebastian (and all of his attachments) and held him high in the air above the bed. Someone else rolled the bed away and moved the rocking chair into its place.

I sat in the chair, and the nurse lowered Sebastian carefully into my arms, without ever having to unhook anything.

Here's a very strong memory that illustrates how the power of touch helped me. It was in the back of the ambulance at the Castlegar airport. Sebastian needed to be airlifted to Vancouver immediately. It was December, and a storm was approaching. The flying doctor refused to let Sebastian fly unless he was intubated. (If he went into distress in the air, inserting a tube in a moving plane would be dangerous.) It was an extremely stressful situation for everyone. I stood at the foot of the stretcher. I wasn't able to touch Sebastian, but I was as close as possible. There was a nurse in the ambulance with us. She stood behind me, and placed her hand gently and firmly on my low back. She kept that gentle pressure there while the tube was placed. (The tube didn't go in easily, and my distress was almost unbearable. I couldn't let it show, though, or I would not have been permitted to stay.) I remember so strongly that loving, caring touch that grounded me and kept me from falling apart so I could continue to be there for my child.

What words of wisdom do I have for parents in similar situations? Be aware of what you want, and what your child needs, and ask for it—again and again. You might not get it—sometimes for really good reasons—but ask. No one knows better than you how to soothe your child. For example, during an early hospital admission, I crawled into Sebastian's little crib and slept there, curled around him. Needless to say, I got no sleep at all for several days, until a caring nurse noticed what I was doing and asked if I wanted Sebastian to have a regular bed! If I'd known better, I would have asked for a bed days earlier.

If you want to hold your child, ask for that. If you want to stay with your child, ask for that. Many times I was advised to leave the room while Sebastian had a painful procedure done. I realize the nurses were trying to spare me distress, but leaving the room was not what I needed, and it definitely wasn't what Sebastian needed. I am grateful now I didn't leave him when he needed me."
—Ellen

I'm so grateful for Ellen's story. This was a family with a long history with me. Ellen was a hands-on mom who taught her two older boys the power of touch to soothe the pain and suffering of their little brother. *Birthing in Good Hands* is for parents like Ellen as they learn to bring relief and refreshment to any situation, whether as light as ushering a new life into the world, or as dark as the loss of life. These are the life transitions I most want to teach people to help using the power of touch.

6

Breasts at Work

Massaging Nursing Breasts

At the moment of conception, breasts change their job description. They instantly graduate from their endearing purpose of attraction to highly functional milking machines. They have a newfound, full-time job of providing life-sustaining food for the newborn. Now the breasts need the attention required for any other hardworking instrument.

The breasts are made of lymphatic nodes, milk ducts, adipose tissue, connective tissue, and the mammary lobules that are milk-producing glands. All this breast structure is housed between the pectoral muscles. The lymphatic system, which helps fight infection and rid the body of wastes, does not contain its own pump, so it relies on the movement of muscles to keep lymphatic fluid moving through the body. As there are no muscles within the breasts themselves, massage becomes even more important for healthy breasts.

Early signs of the breasts needing massaging are an unusual firmness or touch sensitivity. When the breasts get hard, massage, combined with hot and cold hydrotherapy, will relieve the early symptoms of engorgement.

Breast Massage at Every Stage

Breast massage often gets left to the last trimester, but there is no reason for this delay. Start as soon as the mom gets pregnant. Breast massage is an important part of prenatal, postnatal, remedial, and preventative measures. I teach pregnant women to massage their own breasts as well as teaching their partners to do the breast massage. In addition, I always like to teach any other members of the birthing team. Then everyone is prepared for whatever is up the road.

During pregnancy, breast massage helps the breasts grow comfortably without stretch marks, skin tears, or muscle strain. As the breasts change size, the dynamic of the mom's shoulders will also change, usually not for the better. Breast massages during pregnancy can help work out the tight spots and tension areas. Frequency is key: make sure the mom has lots of short massages to keep her posture straight and her tension down. After the baby is born, we have the focus of keeping the breasts working well with a combination of breast massage and hydrotherapy. I advocate continuous breast massaging from pregnancy to well into the first year of breastfeeding.

Throughout my maternity massage career, I have always ensured that my massage oils are edible. On breasts that are feeding an infant, this practice is even more important, just in case of any incidental ingestion. I use grapeseed oil and coconut oil for their superior nutritional values.

Timing

In the first trimester, do breast massage every week; in the second trimester, twice a week; and in the third trimester, once a day.

The massage frequency changes once breasts are producing milk. Especially during the first week of breastfeeding, when the flow of milk varies widely, the breasts need to be massaged all the time and at all times of the day and night. The different stages of milk flow in the first week are helped enormously by breast massage once, twice, or three times a day. Massaging in the morning first thing, massaging before and after feeding, and massaging before and after a daily cold breast wrap are all perfect times to massage. You can read how to do the wrap on page 127 of this chapter.

Post-birth breast massage is meant to be restorative and rejuvenating. It will help immediately in the first hours of the baby's nursing life. Whether it is a five-minute massage or longer, it is easy to employ a few massage strokes. Massaging the breasts can also be part of the couple's recovery program. Any sensual or amorous activity will provide a much-needed holiday for the working breasts!

Broadening the Team

Self-massage plays an important role in nursing breasts. The mom can easily integrate some pre- and postnursing massages for her own breasts. With any needed breast massage, as with breastfeeding problems, women naturally take care of the issue themselves, not ever thinking to include their partners or others. They can tell immediately what kind of pressure is good and where their sore spots are. They can do it in any private location.

However, breast massages don't have to be for her alone. I try to get the whole family involved in learning to massage the nursing breasts. The better the prenatal massage team is at breast massage, the less intimidated they will be when it comes to massaging working breasts that leak all over them.

We are not good at asking our partners or friends to massage us at the best of times, even if all we need is a foot or shoulder rub. But when we're asking someone to touch a part of our body normally associated with sexual attraction, we are even more reluctant. Many women don't like the idea of getting their breasts massaged by someone other than themselves or their partner. However,

if you can take the point of view that asking for help from your partner or friends is another way to allow them into your intimate circle of care and make them feel part of this life changing process, you might see it differently.

After all, breasts have a dual purpose. While our culture celebrates them as an element of sexual attraction, they also have a more down-to-earth purpose: providing the best possible nourishment for newborns. As such, I encourage women to overcome their modesty and seek extra help to ensure their breasts are well cared for; this care will ensure both their own and their baby's well-being. In my experience, mothers are very determined to get their baby the best nutrition possible, and pain is the great eraser of modesty. It has a way of designing efficiency and instantly curing procrastination. Women who are extremely reluctant to ask for help or massage before their baby's birth will willingly demand massage from anyone who can make their pain go away or who can ensure their baby gets the nutrition it needs.

Navigating the politics of the breasts can be tricky. When I shot my film demonstrating breast massage with my patients Holly and Rob, we had many discussions about how to show the massage without attracting creepy Internet traffic. It's unfortunate that we had to spend so much time figuring out how to teach this important skill while dodging unwanted attention. In the end, we settled on a bikini-clad video for general consumption, plus a topless film accessible only to students in my classes.

In the final trimester and postpartum, a thorough breast massage will include large scooping strokes from the armpit to the center of the breast. If you are only doing self-massage for your breasts it will be a bit hard to include your armpit in your routine. This is when it's helpful to have others who can assist. But don't wait until you have a problem to involve others. Make breast massage a normal part of the massage routine.

Some women would rather get a professional to massage their breasts than they would ask a friend or extended family member. When I was studying massage over forty years ago, we were not allowed to massage the breasts for any reason. Luckily, times have changed and breast massage is mandatory training for treatment of maternity symptoms in Canadian professional massage therapy curriculums.

So while professional massage therapists can certainly help you through any breast problem, the power still lies in the hands of family and friends, who are there in the middle of the night to help with painful clogged milk ducts, engorgements, or mastitis. Moms can get better faster and babies will thrive more quickly if everyone learns how to do the massage treatments of these common conditions.

I worked with a young couple having their first baby together, although it was the mother's second child. Four days after the delivery, she ended up with a set of painful breasts. After an emergency call, I taught the newborn's eleven-year-old sister, Maya, the husband, and the mother-in-law to massage and soothe Nikki's engorged breasts.

The massage I taught the first night of Nikki's breast engorgement was repeated the next morning along with a cold breast wrap. Maya was very confident and surpassed the dad in a relaxed approach—very nonchalant, very adaptable. She was my youngest student and yet a great partner in tandem breast massage. She continues her massage skills today by treating her grandmother's broken arm and her daily aches and pains.

This experience taught me to include the whole family in breast massage lessons early, before the delivery. The faster the condition remedies itself, the faster the breasts heal and the faster everyone calms down. This experience was an excellent example of the benefits of extending the massage team beyond the couple. See page 170 for links to some of my video resources for breast massage, as well as other aspects of maternity massage.

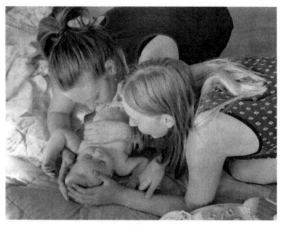

Figure 6.1. Nikki and Maya (who was just eleven years old when she learned to massage her pregnant mom).

"Christine and I were with mom during her labor, massaging her back. Using Christine's powerful knowledge, we were able to keep her breathing at a normal pace and take some of the pressure off of her back and shoulders. After quite a few hours with little progress, the doctor broke her water. My mother went from four centimeters' dilation to full-on baby in just over two hours. I was able to go and sit right beside the doctor, right in the action." —Maya

"A couple of days after the birth of my son, my milk came in and I was SO engorged and in so much pain. Christine taught my daughter and I how to do a breast massage and towel wrap. She got a bath towel wet with cold water and wrapped both breasts in a figure-eight pattern. She did this a few times. While the cold towel was helping with the pain and inflammation, she showed us how to massage the breasts and how to use ice cubes massaged in a circular motion. The pain and discomfort were dramatically reduced by the next day. It was truly a lifesaver, and I believe it was the reason I didn't end up with mastitis, or any further complications." —Nikki

Hydrotherapy for Breast Health

Hydrotherapy can be used in combination with massage for many conditions, but it is particularly useful for breast health. Following are some of the techniques I use and teach most frequently.

Cold breast wrap

I often use a cold breast wrap at the beginning of a face-up pregnancy or postpartum massage routine. The application of icy cold to the breasts encourages blood to rush to the surface of the skin, creating better circulation and healing for any problems. While the breasts are wrapped in cold towels, I do the rest of the massage (arms, legs, abdomen, etc.). That way, my breast massage routine will be a warm contrast to the cold wrap. The daily application of a cold breast wrap can also be a soothing way to let the mom nap while her body responds to the hydrotherapy.

The breast wrap is done with a towel large enough to wrap around both breasts in a figure eight. A towel that is highly absorbent with good cotton fiber will hold the water well and keep it in reserve.

1. Soak the towel in cold water.
2. Wring it out so the towel is wet but not dripping. Keep the towel as cold as possible while getting it from the source to the mother. For example, keep it folded; do not extend it until right before you wrap the breasts so the towel does not have a chance to heat up.
3. Wrap the breasts with a big lift along the bottom of the breasts and up along the sides toward the armpits. Wrap the towel from underneath the breasts up and around the top so the ends of the towel meet at the sternum or breastbone.
4. Now unfold the towel over any exposed skin so the breasts are totally covered with cold, wet towel.
5. Wrap a large plastic garbage bag over the wrap to seal out the air. We want the impact of the cold to be as powerful as possible. The cold stimulates circulation in the breast, causing a rush of blood to the area and increased warmth.
6. Place a dry towel over the wrap and tuck it under the mom's sides to secure and insulate the wrap. Follow this with a warm blanket for further insulation. You want the breasts to reheat through their own circulation, not the outside air temperature. This increased circulation will help the breasts heal faster.

Figure 6.2. Cold breast wrap.

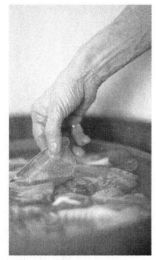

a. Soak a towel in ice water.

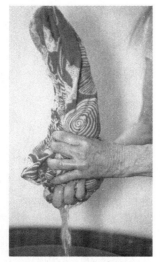

b. Wring out enough of the water that it isn't dripping, but keep it as wet as possible.

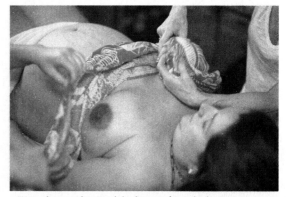

c. Wrap the towel around the breasts from the bottom.

(Continued, next page)

Figure 6.2. Cold breast wrap, continued.

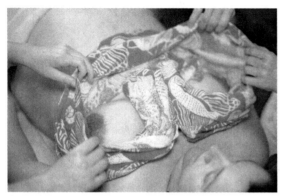

d. Wrap the towel up the sides and down the front so each breast is circled.

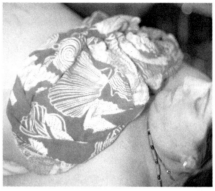

e. Spread the towel so the breasts are completely covered in cold towel.

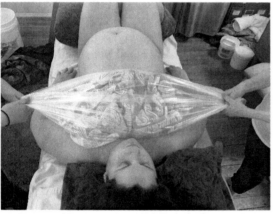

f. Cover the cold towel with a plastic garbage bag as insulation.

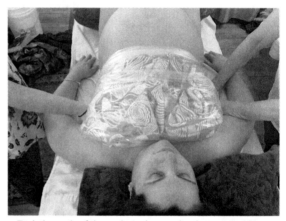

g. Tuck the ends of the garbage bag under the mom's sides securely.

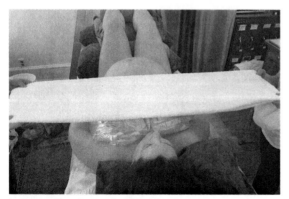

h. Cover with a dry towel and tuck in.

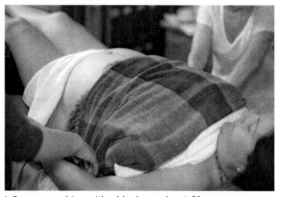

i. Cover everything with a blanket and wait fifteen to twenty minutes before removing the wraps and beginning the breast massage.

Keep the wrap on the breasts while you continue with other parts of the massage. The towel usually takes about five minutes to heat up. The body's natural heating process will take about ten minutes to peak. By then, the body will warm up past where it was before you applied the cold wrap, causing sweating and detoxification. After fifteen to twenty minutes, once you've finished all the massage you can do with the mom in a supine position, remove the wrap and finish off with a breast massage.

If the breasts do not feel warm when you remove the wrap, you either did not wrap them tightly enough or insulate your wrap well enough. Either way, usually outside air getting in is the culprit here. Even a cool wrap provides some hydrotherapeutic benefit, but if you can, do the wrap again if the mom does not heat up in twenty minutes.

Ice massage

I use ice massage with any engorgement or clogged or blocked milk ducts. Use an ice popsicle or an ice cube edge in place of your fingers to massage around the breast perimeter in a figure eight with small, circular kneading strokes. This is a duplication of the normal breast massage routine, but using the ice instead of your fingers.

Be careful to not overstay your welcome. Frequency needs enthusiasm, so don't use ice massage too long in any one session. As the skin numbs, it is easy to keep going because the relief is so welcome. But instead of continuing it is better to come back an hour later and do it again.

Cold hands breast massage

Fill a bucket or bowl with crushed ice. Massage the ice with both your hands until you can't stand it or your fingers start to go numb or both. Repeat this process two or three times during the breast massage to keep your hands as cold as possible. You want the breasts to heat up from their own circulation, not from your warming hands. Increased circulation promotes faster healing and relief from pain.

Snow packs

Fill a resealable plastic bag with snow. Usually the medium-sized bags work best. Flatten the snow inside the bag to create a compress about a quarter of an inch thick. Apply to the breast wherever the most congestion has occurred. Where the pain is greatest, the ice is most needed.

Hot water bottles

Two to four hot water bottles can provide portable hydrotherapy. All four bottles can be used at once with the same or contrasting temperatures of water. Make sure the bottles are not plum full so they will mold to the breast and make greater, more effective skin contact.

Where to apply them varies with the breast condition. If the mom is comfortable with her arms above her head, then the water bottles can lie in her armpits and alongside the breasts.

If the mom has her arms by her sides, then hot water bottles can easily insert between her arms and the sides of her body. This method will heat or cool both sides of the body at once, as well as the sides of her breasts. I will usually refresh the hot water bottles during my massages, heating them up again or cooling them down, whichever is required.

Contrast bathing

The symptoms of engorgement and overactive nursing breasts can be relieved with contrasting temperatures from a handheld or wall-mounted showerhead. Start with warm to warmer water and then change to cool and cold. Each time you contrast, make the difference more extreme. Do the contrast at least five times and always end with cold for the most long-lasting effect.

Contrast hot and cold applications

Follow the instructions for the cold breast wrap, but alternate between applications of cold towels and hot towels. Place a towel in each of two buckets. Pour ice water in one bucket and keep a kettle simmering to keep the other filled with hot water.

Apply the towel from one of the buckets to the breasts, while the other towel is preparing in the other bucket. Insulate the wrap as you learned for the cold breast wraps. Alternate temperatures at least four times.

Hot Epsom salt wraps

Add at least a cup of Epsom salt to a bucket of hot water. Let a towel soak in the hot Epsom water and wring it out lightly. You want it wet, but not sopping. Wrap the breasts quickly, insulate your wrap with plastic wrap or a plastic garbage bag, and then wrap with another blanket or towel to trap the heat. After about twenty minutes, wash the breasts with cold and then warm water. I recommend doing this wrap at least once a week, even if the mom doesn't have any problems with her breasts. If the mom does have problems, you can remove the breast wrap, do the massage, and then do another wrap.

Breast Massage for Nursing Breasts

Breast massage is an important part of the full-body massage routine for pregnant women, long before nursing begins. But once the breasts are nursing instead of pregnant, you may need to include more hydrotherapy in your breast care routine. I recommend one or more cold breast wraps per day, especially in the first weeks. If the mom is experiencing any breast discomfort, you may also want to prepare a bowl of ice water for cold hand massaging. A quick summary of the breast massage steps follow. For more details, review pages 49–51.

Common Problems During Breastfeeding

My own breast massages during my pregnancy helped me prevent stretch marks and got me more comfortable with my new breasts. However, years of professional practice have given me invaluable experience with all sorts of common day-to-day issues that occur with breastfeeding moms.

BREAST MASSAGE SUMMARY MENU

1. Apply a cold breast wrap to the breasts.
2. Do a head, neck, and shoulder massage while breasts are cooling.
3. Place a hot water bottle under the neck after the head, neck, and shoulder massage. Reserve a second bottle to place on the breastbone (sternum) at the end of the treatment.
4. Effleurage to the breasts from above the head or from the side of the mom.
5. Scooping the breast in upward alternating hands moving toward each other.
6. Fingertip kneading to the attachments of the pectoral muscles (along the breastbone, and out to the attachment at the armpit).
7. Scooping to the axilla (only if the mom has a problem with overproduction, in which case you should have a milk bottle handy!) Use a C-shape to your hand to alternate scooping to the armpit. Work in both directions: up to down and down to up along the side of the body at the armpit.
8. Fingertip kneading all around the breasts in a figure-eight pattern. Keep the pressure of each stroke upward (never pulling downward on the breast).
9. Scooping the breasts (going back to the general introductory strokes).
10. Effleurage to finish.
11. Place the second hot water bottle on the mom's sternum.

Milk production

Many women experience milk production problems, whether underproduction or overproduction. Both can cause anxiety and stress for the mom and other members of the household. I use the same basic massage techniques for either concern.

For overproduction, massage helps drain tight, engorged breasts. Keep bottles handy to freeze extra milk for future use or to donate to a milk bank. Eventually massage will help the flow of milk even out.

For underproduction, the more you massage and milk the breast, the more milk will be

Levels of milk production are unpredictable, just as the timing for your milk coming in can be unpredictable. Keeping happy and relaxed can help milk production, but staying stress-free in the early days home with a newborn can be a challenge, especially if the house is full of visiting relatives. Put extra guests to work on massage to make them part of the solution, not the problem.

stimulated to flow. Massage, by promoting relaxation and release of the hormone oxytocin, can increase milk production in breastfeeding mothers.[10] I encourage moms struggling with underflow to massage their breasts as much as possible.

Hydrotherapy can also help. Ice massage is one of the most successful additions to the breast massage routine for increasing milk production. Use an ice popsicle or you can hold an ice cube with a facecloth and do your figure-eight kneading around the breasts with the ice instead of your fingers. Alternate between ice massage and hot water bottles, hot towels, hot packs, or heated beanbags. The contrasting temperatures provide circulatory stimulation, which will increase production quickly.

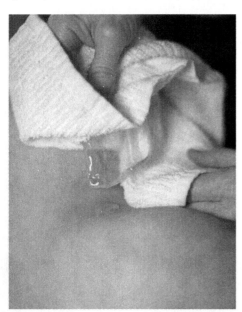

Figure 6.3. Wipe up any drips from melting ice with the towel.

You can do the massage and hydrotherapy combination several times a day if the mom finds it helpful. The application of massage will warm up the breast as it increases the circulation. The ice-cold hand massage technique will also provide good contrast for this underproduction problem.

Having the baby snuggled between the breasts for skin-on-skin contact also helps encourage milk flow, as does playing music while you nurse. During the 1970s, playing music for cows was found to increase milk production by three percent. In humans, playing soothing music such as classical or country has similar benefits. So snuggle with your baby between your breasts after breastfeeding and breast massaging, continue to play the favorite massage music you used in pregnancy massage, and look forward to that three percent increase flowing into your welcoming breasts!

Painful nipples

Breastfeeding should feel good. But that feeling good quickly becomes not-so-good if the nipples become problematic. Cracked, bleeding, or blistered nipples can be excruciating.

Once the nipples are blistered, you will need fast solutions to soothe the area and bring down the inflammation as quickly as possible. Hydrotherapy in combination with massage will give you the best and quickest results for any cracks or sores on the nipples. The contrast of hot and cold temperatures helps flush the vascular system and speed up the recovery time.

Bringing fresh blood to an area that needs to heal is a basic premise of massage therapy. Doing the basic breast massage will help, but as always, avoid all nipple contact. Massage each breast for about ten minutes. Interrupt the open "c" scooping of the breast about every two minutes for some effleurage and figure-eight fingertip kneading.

Some oils—calendula, olive, and comfrey—are good for repairing, strengthening, and softening nipples that may become cracked and sore in the early stages of breastfeeding.

Direct ice massage to the nipple stimulates blood circulation at the same time as providing pain relief. I encourage my nursing moms to use ice directly on blistered nipples, gently massaging around the nipple and areola with facecloth wrapped around three ice cubes or with an ice popsicle. I even recommend this ice massage to new moms before they develop nipple problems.

Another old-fashioned remedial and preventive measure for painful nipples is "air bathing." This is simply giving the breasts no confinement, exposing them to the air without any kind of covering. I also use this method with my palliative patients and babies with a variety of diaper rashes.

Breasts needing air bathing usually do best with the breasts up; not hanging down. Flip them up for air bathing where the sun doesn't shine! Lying down is usually the easiest method for accomplishing this. If possible, go braless while the rash or sore persists. You might also use some of the baby's zinc ointment directly on the sore patch to speed the healing.

If possible, expose the breasts to the sun to further encourage healing. Build up exposure from under a minute to three minutes over the first five days. Then do five minutes daily. This not only helps condition the entire breast and nipple, but it also helps to fight infection and dry up any cracking.

Breast massage is useful to increase milk production and prevent clogged ducts, breast engorgement, and mastitis. For as long as women have been breastfeeding, breast massage has been an effective insurance against these potential problems. Patients referred to me with problems from engorgement to problems of not enough milk have the same solution: massage therapy.

Baby Massage Basics

Common baby conditions such as constipation, gas, teething, and respiratory coughs and colds can also be treated with massage, as can more unusual conditions such as infantile torticollis. Massaging your baby daily will give you a larger skill set to induce sleep and soothe times of discomfort and irritability and at the same time will forge strong parental bonds.

Parents make the best massage therapists for their infants. You can be hands on, whatever the time of the day. You are invested in your newborn's well-being. Whether your child has the natural aches and pains of a growing newborn or is a special needs baby, massage is a huge investment in your child's health and growth.

The Arrival Massage

We are held in a womb of close contact for our first nine months. Massage can help continue that warmth and tactility after birth.

Babies who arrive through C-section miss the uterine contractions and big squeeze of vaginal birth. We can help these babies by massaging them to simulate that first massage. Massages performed in the labor room are highly effective for strengthening respiratory and circulatory functioning. Massage is certainly a kinder, gentler replacement for the old-fashioned slap to start a newborn breathing!

Babies with special deliveries, such as delayed births with delayed breathing, lack of oxygen, or a baby in distress in utero, can be helped with immediate massage. Despondent, non-responsive babies have traditionally been stimulated with cold water or massage, skin stimulation that saved their lives. In a recent delivery I attended, the baby arrived lifeless, showing no movement or breathing, but with immediate rubbing by the attending physician, the baby came to life.

Babies who arrive with the uterine massage well done, which means they had the contracting massage from the mother's body in labor, are still perfect candidates for an arrival massage. Even babies with an easy delivery need to have their little feet rubbed to get their peripheral circulation up and running. It is great to watch those tiny blue feet turn pink!

If possible, I like to do the back, legs, and foot massage when the baby is lying on the mother. The baby never needs to be off the mother's body for this first massage.

Lubricate your fingertips and palms (or the other parent's) with coconut oil—it's the best nourishment for this new skin. The most important thing for the arrival massage is skin-to-skin contact. Skin contact is good for the baby and the new parents. That intimacy and bonding is needed in the first hour of delivering the child, and the effect is soothing for all parties, including any siblings in attendance.

A hands-on parenting style is started with touch in the first minutes of the baby's life. This touch strengths the life-support systems of respiration, digestion, and neurological functioning. The affection and love for your children expressed through massage is an outlet worth devoting time to every day.

Failure to Thrive

When thriving is a concern, massage is a good therapy to increase the baby's weight, as medical research now supports. Research suggests that certain brain chemicals released by touch, or others released in its absence, may be responsible for some infants' failure to thrive.[11]

Each baby that is not thriving is different—not all causes stem from lack of touch. However, no matter what the cause, I recommend increasing the frequency of massages from once to three times a day. Babies who are not thriving should be passed around, held, and handled. These loving-touches are the best way to increase appetite and promote baby well-being. With my barnyard experience, I know that the mammals of this world thrive best with tactility at its highest.

BABY MASSAGE MENU

Below is a baby massage routine I use in my practice and teaching. Basically there are no mistakes about where to start and where to end. If the baby has a particular problem, you might want to address the problem with it. Or just the opposite, it might be advantageous to address the problem by starting peripherally and work toward the center of the issue. Either way, you will develop your own sequence, but I encourage you to vary your style and not get stuck in just one approach.

1. **Back massage:** Gets everything affected through the central nervous system.
2. **Legs (posterior):** gluteals, hamstrings, and lower legs and feet.
3. **Anterior trunk:** abdomen (digestive) and chest (respiratory).
4. **Leg pumping for digestion.**
5. **Arms.**
6. **Legs (anterior).**
7. **Face and scalp, including the jaw.**

Beginning the Massage

The main difference between adult and baby massage is that babies are constantly moving so you need to adapt your strokes to move with them. Other than that, the classification of strokes is identical and the treatment of most everyday conditions, from constipation to respiratory problems, is also similar with a few adaptations.

Never pull or push a baby's joint when he or she resists. Always work with the baby's movement.

Before you start massaging your baby, arrange a warm, draft-free area with lots of towels and toys. Remove all jewelry and cover yourself with towels or an apron to protect your clothes from oil stains.

Place the baby on a towel in front of you. The baby can be

- **Supine:** lying face up on its back
- **Prone:** tummy down with the head turned to one side and legs either extended or tucked in
- **Side-lying:** between your hands in a comfort sandwich. Have one hand on the tummy and one hand on the back. Try hooking the upper leg of the baby over your arm so it is secure.

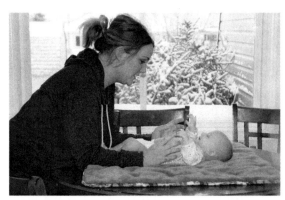

Figure 7.1. Place the baby on a soft blanket or towel. You can turn the whole towel to get at the baby's other side.

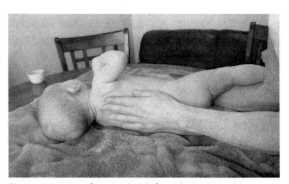

Figure 7.2. A comfort sandwich for side-lying position.

Some babies respond to side-lying better than face-up or face-down massages. If the baby has a tendency to have a favored side, turn the head to the disfavored side so it can stretch out the neck and re-establish a balance. This is done by having the tight side of the neck in the downward position and then the "lazy" side will tighten to resist the side that is kinked and contracted.

The side-lying position is also good for babies that need drainage for the lungs. This is important for mid-lobe drainage for babies needing respiratory attention in the first few hours or older babies who have ongoing respiratory issues. Again, you massage on both sides for balance.

To begin, choose the position the baby seems most comfortable in. Oil your hands and slowly rub them together to warm them. Use a natural oil, such as almond or coconut, because they are well-absorbed by the skin.

"Why massage babies? Massaging at a young age creates an incredible closeness and bond; for my son and daughter, it gave them an understanding of close tender touch. Today, both are very willing to be close and use their hands to show affection. I think this comes from the early massaging they got in our family. In teenagehood, it was a bond. There's nothing my teenagers liked better than having their feet rubbed. It also spurred on discussions that weren't happening otherwise. I found that while I rubbed their feet, they became more open about what was going on in their lives."
—Sydnee

Massaging after a morning bath, when the baby is fresh and warm, starts the day the right way for both parties, babies and massagers! Or you can use the bath after a massage to further the relaxation. I massage my granddaughter and then I fill the sink and let her float in the warm water, filling the sink every five minutes with warmer water. She sleeps like a log after that combo!

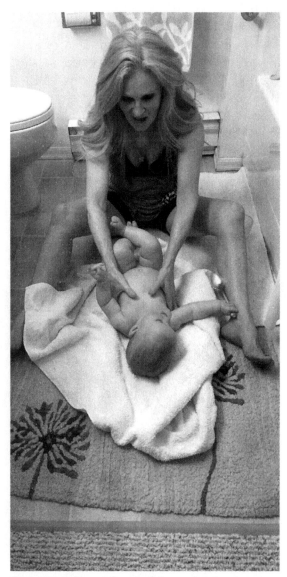

Figure 7.3. Before or after a bath is a perfect time to massage your baby.

I used to massage Crystal in the car before a lunch date, and then without fail she would sleep throughout the entire meal. It doesn't matter if you massage through the baby's clothing. While skin-to-skin contact is important for early bonding, it's the significance of touch that matters in the long term. Most of us have a memory of the significance of touch in our lives, and it usually is not a naked touch, skin on skin, but rather a comforting gesture, a reassuring back pat, or a hug.

BABY MASSAGE IN AN UPRIGHT POSITION

In addition to teaching prone, supine, and side-lying positions for massage, I teach new parents how to massage babies in an upright posture to give them every possible way to start their routine and keep the baby comfortable. Some babies find the prone or supine positions unsettling. The upright massage can be done with the baby in a snuggly against the parents as they are "wearing" the baby or seated on your lap or another surface. Newborns to toddlers can be massaged in a seated position.

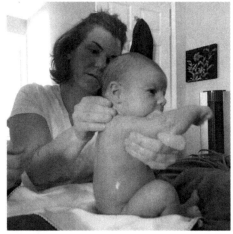

Figure 7.4. To use an upright position for massaging your baby, hold it securely with one hand and massage with the other.

Although the back massage is the most obvious for this posture, you can actually do the entire massage routine with the baby in an upright posture. While older babies and toddlers can be self-supporting, for newborns you will need to support the baby with one hand and massage with the other.

All the strokes, including effleurage, kneading, and wringing, can be adapted to use one hand. For example, instead of massaging with alternate thumb kneading, you will just use single-handed thumb kneading. When the baby is seated, you can use the same techniques for massaging under the hip that you use to work under adults. Just lever your fingers up against whatever surface the baby is sitting on to massage under the hip and into the gluteals. Just be sure to work both sides of the baby's body, changing their position to allow you to switch hands.

For digestive massage, place one hand on the tummy and the other hand on the back. Move the hand on the abdomen in a clockwise direction and the hand on the back counterclockwise. While one hand is at the top of the abdomen, the other is at the bottom of the back.

As an alternative to the one-handed technique, you can get someone to hold the baby in a seated position and perform the classical sequence and technique. In my classes, I have one student holding the baby at the back or sides as I teach parents the tandem massage.

When babies are newborn it may seem counterintuitive to use an upright position for massage, but with a baby in a snuggly, held against the chest or on your lap, babies can be well-supported with no strain on their neck. They can curl into their birthing position and you can do their massage without the prone or supine positions.

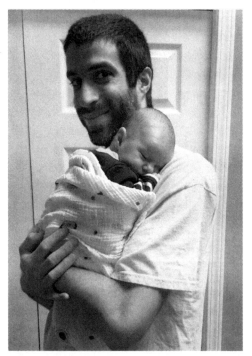

Figure 7.5. The upright position is perfect for both parents and babies—it can also be skin to skin. Walking, bouncing, and jiggling are great add-ons to the back massage movements. Most importantly, this adaptation facilitates massaging anywhere and everywhere, home or hospital.

Back Massage

Choose a position your baby seems comfortable in:

- Prone, with the baby lying on its tummy
- Side-lying, with one hand on the tummy to stabilize while the other hand massages the back
- Seated, supporting the baby with a hand across the tummy or shoulders from the side of the baby. If the baby is old enough to be self-supporting in an upright position, the massage can be done with two hands working up and down the back.

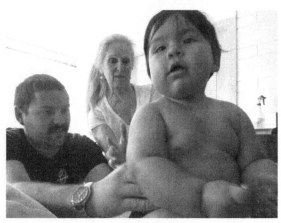

Figure 7.6. Once the baby is old enough to sit up, you can massage the back with both hands on. Give the low back a massage in a seated position with the hands wrapping around the baby's hips. This gives the thumbs lots of room to massage the middle of the back where the erector spinae run the length of the baby's back. This dad has large hands that could easily accomplish this two-handed back massage.

As with adults, use the basic principle of moving from general to specific and then general strokes.

1. **Effleurage:** Use the entire palmar surface of your hands, including your fingers, to effleurage from the bottom up or top down:
   - **Bottom up:** Move up the back from the sacrum to shoulders along the erector spinae that run parallel to the spine. Glide with pressure on the way up to the top of the shoulders, wrap around the trapezius muscles and out to the top of the arms (the deltoids), and then glide down the sides of the baby to the starting position.
   - **Top down:** Start at the shoulders and glide down the erector spinae, being careful not to put pressure on the spine itself. When you get to the sacrum, circle your hands to the baby's sides and pull them up to the shoulders, out to the deltoids, over the trapezius, and back to the starting position.

You can do both styles of effleurage in the same sequence. Sometimes I do one version at the beginning of the massage and then end with the other version.

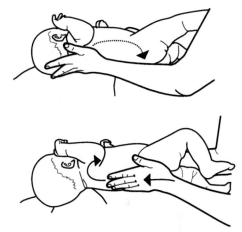

Figure 7.7. Sandwich the baby between your hands to perform your effleurage from neck down and around and back up.

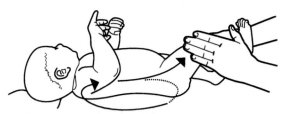

Figure 7.8. You can also effleurage from the lower back up to the shoulders, wrapping around and coming back down the leg.

2. **Petrissage:** All these strokes use alternating pressure with palms, thumbs, and fingertips.
   - **Wringing:** This is a full-handed stroke that covers the entire back at once (bilateral) or half the back at a time (unilateral). Pull

one hand and push your other hand across the back with enough pressure to cause the skin to twist between the hands. Then reverse directions to wring the other way. The hands must wrap around the sides of the baby's back to be thorough. If you want, you can change to unilateral wringing, just doing the baby's back on the side closest to you and the side farthest away from you separately. Then go back to bilateral wringing to put both sides together again. I like to also wring the top of the shoulders with a wringing stroke up and over the top of the trapezius muscles. The shoulder wringing stroke is excellent for babies with forceps deliveries or wryneck.

- **Palmar kneading**: This is done with one palm, stacked palms (reinforced), or both palms moving independently (simultaneous). Whether the stroke is heading up or down the back, the direction of pressure for each kneading stroke is up and away from the spine. About four or five palmar kneading strokes are applied on either side of the spine.

- **Alternate thumb kneading**: With small, overlapping circles, move your alternating thumbs up the erector spinae muscles from the sacrum to the base of the skull. The pressure is up and out without picking up your thumbs—they stay attached to the skin at all times. Move your thumb kneading up and down the back in columns on either side of the spine.

  Linger longer in any spots of concern. For example, if the baby has digestive problems, give extra strokes to the mid to low back area, where the nerves that supply the digestive organs exit the spine. If respiration is a problem, do more alternate thumb kneading along the thorax. For babies without any specific concern, I tend to massage the erector spinae and neck, and then spend a little extra time on the low back working along the upper edges of the hips (iliac crest).

- **Fingertip kneading**: Use single-handed or reinforced, straight fingers, putting the pressure of each stroke up and away from the spine in a line of about ten overlapping strokes along the erector spinae from the base of the skull to the sacrum.

Figure 7.9. Baby back wringing.

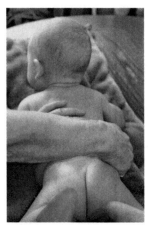

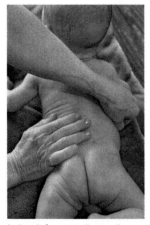

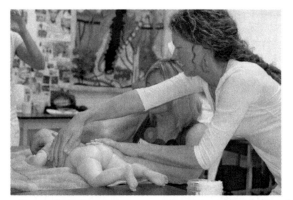

a. When wringing, be sure to get your hands right around the baby's sides to cover the whole back thoroughly.

b. Don't forget to "marry" your hands so they move close by each other.

c. Parents learn best in one-to-one tutorials with a "hands-on" methodology in which the therapist puts her hands on the parent's hands or has the parent put her hands on the therapist's hands. This method allows the parent to feel the appropriate rhythm and pressure. Here Sarah Yarwood, a birth doula, teaches grandbaby massage using the "hands on my hands" approach to learning wringing.

3. **Tapotement**: Use gentle, percussive rhythmic movements to help stimulate the thorax and aid in expectoration, or simply to stimulate circulation in the baby's back.

   - **Loose fingertip hacking**: Flick the fingertips with the hands moving quickly up and down in a side position.
   - **Stiff fingertip hacking**: Make a chopping motion with the hands acting as one, brushing by each other as they move.
   - **Cupping**: Use a curved hand to tap around the back, making a hollow sound.
   - **Beating**: Use a flattened fist with a loose-wristed motion up and down.
   - **Pounding**: Make tight fists so that there is a cushion at the little finger side of your hand and pound gently with a rolling action toward yourself—not an up and down motion. Use gentle strokes along the erector spinae.

4. **Fingertip kneading, alternate thumb kneading, and palmar kneading**: Finish the massage by moving back out to the more general strokes. You may also want to add a few effleurages.

5. **Light reflex stroking**: This is the final stroke, brushing the fingertips lightly along the spine.

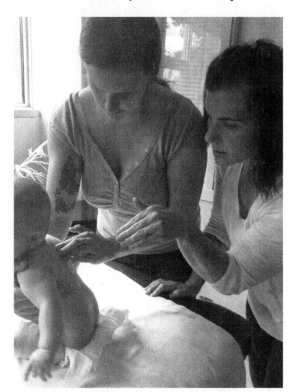

Figure 7.10. Tracy, a doula, demonstrates a baby back and neck massage using a hands-on methodology.

Massage for the Extremities

The arms and legs in the baby massage routine follow the same principles as the adult version. The principle of "uncorking the bottle" is also applied to the tiny human in front of you. Undo any tension in the upper aspect of the extremity and then focus on what is below that level. Where the arm and leg hook into the trunk of the body is an intersection of elaborate structures. The muscles, bones, and joints are hard-working and, in the case of a newborn, still evolving.

The baby's hip joints and shoulder joints, in particular, are still soft and unstable in the first few months, as they are not fully formed. They are growing to accommodate the job they have to do in the future of this person's life: holding them up. Those joints have our attention in the first couple of years of the child's life as he or she learns to stand, then walk.

For this reason, I don't use any pulling motions on the extremities. For instance, when I do a digestive treatment and I use leg pumping, I make sure that the angle of the movement is in line with the joint itself.

In this phase of newborn development, babies need massage as their body changes and develops their systems of muscular strength and endurance. My granddaughter, Paige, was a "runner" at seven months. Her legs were always in a highland fling, whether eating or plotting her next endearing moment. In her daily massage before bed, she had a good massage on those hard-working legs.

MASSAGE TO ENCOURAGE BODY ALIGNMENT

Babies have a natural bow shape to their legs—normally this straightens as they age, but this doesn't always happen.

Sometimes this bow is just genetics, not a deformity per se. I have a patient who is over a year old and her hips are quite unusual. Her legs are very far apart and she has a distinctive bow-legged gait. However, her brother was identical at the same age, with the same gait. Three years later, you would never know he had a bow-legged posture when first walking.

Regardless of the family etiology, it is important to treat the little girl with proper massage therapy to keep loosening any contracted structures. Swimming at an early age will encourage general strengthening. The parents of these two kids are keen to be hands on, tracking the progress of their children's growth, and hoping for a natural resolution to what could be a problem up the road.

If the problem doesn't resolve, my patient could require remedial splinting. Splinting combined with massage can often remedy even severe deformities. The idea is to massage to make the joints as supple as possible, then splint to realign the leg, then massage again upon the removal of the splints to refresh the circulation and help establish the new pattern of leg alignment.

MASSAGE MENU FOR THE ARMS, LEGS, AND NECK

1. **Effleurage**: Three times minimum.
2. **Petrissage**: Wringing, single-handed palmar kneading, reinforced palmar kneading, alternate thumb kneading, single-handed thumb kneading.
3. **Cupping tapotement**.
4. **Light reflex stroking**: Overhanded, simultaneous, wringing, palmar, and back of the hand.
5. **Repeat the introductory strokes**: Effleurage with light reflex stroking.

Arms

1. **Effleurage**: Start at the hand and spread the coconut oil over the arm to the shoulder, wrapping around from the front to the back of the shoulder, and then gliding back down without pressure to the hand again. After you glide back down to the hand, switch hands and do another single-handed effleurage up the arm, this time more focused on the inner arm to the armpit. This is a divided two-handed effleurage, alternating between hands with a loose grip at the baby's wrist.

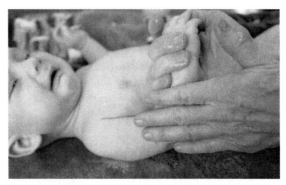

Figure 7.11. The baby's arm will probably be moving the whole time you massage it. This is different from adult massage, where you can control the arm and hold the hand at the wrist. With babies, try to move with their movements. Hold the baby's hand with your inside hand, and with your other hand, do a single-handed effleurage to the outside of the arm.

2. **Palmar kneading to the shoulder**: Single-handed palmar kneading is done with cupped hand circles encompassing the entire tiny shoulder from the front to the back. The "outside" hand does the circles while the other hand loosely holds the baby's hand or wrist.
3. **Thumb kneading to the upper arm**: Now transition to single-handed thumb kneading on the deltoid muscle at the top of the arm and then on the triceps on the back of the upper arm. Then change the position of your hands and do alternate thumb kneading to the biceps, cradling the arm between your hands.
4. **Palmar kneading to the elbow**: Bend the baby's arm, cup the elbow, and circle it with

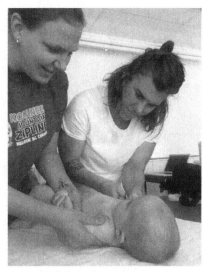

Figure 7.12. Tandem baby massage.

your palm. Do this circling movement at least three times.

5. **Alternate thumb kneading to the lower arm**: Knead the forearm with your thumbs from the inner elbow to the wrist three times. The pressure of your thumbs is always toward the heart. Now do the same movement to the outer forearm.

6. **Alternate thumb kneading to the hand**: When the outer forearm massage is done, move to the back of the hand, spending focused time at the wrist. Now bend the baby's arm at the elbow and bend the wrist back, exposing the ligamentous attachments at the wrist. Here is where I go against my principle of every stroke of pressure being toward the heart. With the wrist bent back, I thumb knead the palm of the hand with alternate movements, kneading from the wrist toward the fingers. This alternate thumb kneading is very different from the grown-up version where the hand stays calm and still under your hands. This little hand will be moving and your hand massage will need to move along with it!

7. **Corkscrew the fingers**: What seems impossible is next: the fingers! Newborn baby fingers are so tiny they seem impossible to massage since they are usually fisted and tight.

However, slow and gentle prying will give you a free finger to wring, one at a time.

Recently, I massaged the toughest little fists I have ever experienced in all my years of baby massage. This little baby held her hands so tightly that she blistered her palms. However, with daily massage over seven months, these same hands are now relaxed and open. This is an example of what daily and twice-daily massages can do if started early enough to change patterns that may have been established before birth. This neurological repatterning required diligent family massage therapy.

8. **Finale**: Finish with light reflex stroking or effleurage.

Legs (anterior)

1. **Effleurage**: Work from the toes to the hip and back to the feet. Move up with pressure, wrapping your hands across the leg and coming back down either side without pressure. Do this three times. The outside hand extends to the upper hip and around the head of the femur.

2. **Fingertip kneading at the hip**: Whether you have the baby's diapers on or off makes no difference. If the diaper is on, get under the elastic and around the hip. This is not just "uncorking the bottle," it is also a good spot to stimulate the digestive system and keep babies comfortable. Mobilizing the hips activates digestion.

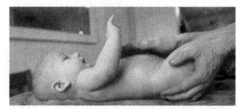

Figure 7.13. As well as working the front of the hip, spend focused time at the back with fingertip kneading on the gluteal muscles, so the hip is lifted up with each kneading stroke. Lever your fingertips up so you are pushing back against the surface the baby is lying on. The baby will lift up and down as your fingertips lever into the hip area. This sounds more dramatic than it appears in real life. It is a concentrated effort to undo tension in the hip and get the hip moving at the same time, opening up the circulation to the entire leg.

Smooth out this hip work with a big general stroke like single-handed palmar kneading. Then we can move on to the rest of the leg, having uncorked that "bottle!"

3. **Wringing to the leg**: Lift the baby's leg straight up and wring the leg with both hands wrapped around it.

Again, remember that this hip joint is not fully formed and stable, so it is important to keep the angle of the leg in line with the hip, not in a "V" shape. As you work on the thigh and the quadriceps, keep a close eye on the alignment of the leg at the knee, watching for bowing or turning tendencies. We want to be hands on observing changes in the legs and especially the position of the knee as the baby grows.

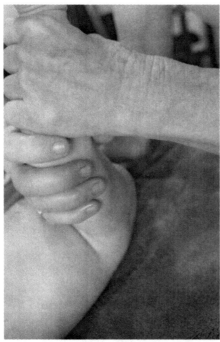

Figure 7.14. This straight-up leg wringing is a style that can't be done with an adult. Wringing up and down the entire leg helps keep the circulation moving and loosens up surface tension.

4. **Alternate thumb kneading to the thigh**: This is a mainstay stroke for the thigh. Do alternate thumb kneading up and down the thigh, following the route of the quadriceps muscles. These muscles are not clearly defined to the touch, so just massage up the front of the thigh from knee to hip. Massage the inner thigh, middle thigh, and outer thigh in three different lines down to the kneecap. I loved teaching my daughter her muscles as she grew up and delighted in her pronunciation of the anatomic name of the kneecap, the patella. Wringing and alternate thumb kneading are the two strokes I use the most on this upper part of the leg.

5. **Knee massage**: This is a favorite massage spot for adults and children alike. The knee is the greatest weight-bearing joint in our body. For this reason, it is the slowest joint to form and strengthen. Unlike barnyard animals, we do not jump up after delivery and run around the field of hope. Instead, we slowly and steadily gain our balance over the first year of our lives. This is an important time for helping that development.

Massaging the knee is important as we don't know what is up ahead for kids in their development. Whether they turn out to have normal legs or specially shaped legs with challenging joints, the knees play an important role in holding the body up, so keeping the legs and knee joints massaged is good insurance for the best growing results.

Use a modified wringing stroke for the knee. House the patella between your hands, one above and one below the kneecap, and slowly wrap around to the back of the baby's leg.

Then use alternate thumb kneading to circle the entire perimeter of the kneecap. Give extra attention to the patellar tendon, the attachment of the lower leg at the bottom of the knee.

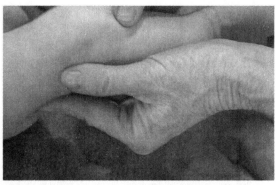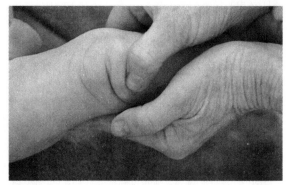

Figure 7.15. Use your thumb to knead around the bottom and sides of the patella.

6. **Lower leg**: In the womb, babies are used to being in a curled-up position. After birth, their arms and legs start to unfurl, and massage helps them unfurl the right way. Pay special attention to the back of the knee, where the muscles from the hamstrings attach on either side the lower leg. These muscles are getting stronger with the newborn's leg movements. You can massage these attachments from the front or the back.

The front of the lower leg has the tibialis anterior that runs from the knee to the foot. This muscle is always moving with baby's reflexes in early infancy. Eventually, it will stabilize the ankle as the baby's foot hits the ground during the contact phase of walking (eccentric contraction) and then it helps pull the foot clear of the ground during the swing phase of walking (concentric contraction). It is a muscle to watch as the baby grows, as it always needs massaging.

Use alternate thumb kneading up and down the tibialis anterior from the outside of the knee to where it inserts into the baby's foot. I do some wringing strokes on the lower leg before and after the alternate thumb kneading.

7. **Thumb kneading around the ankle bones**: Use both of your hands to knead around the tiny ankle bones. This massage works the bumps of muscle attachment on either side of the ankle, the Achilles tendon, and the heel of the foot. Focus your fingertip and thumb kneading at the point where the gastrocnemius muscle attaches to the calcaneus (heel).

8. **Single-handed wringing to the toes**: Cup the baby's heel in one hand and wring each tiny toe from base to tip. Even large dad-fingers can get around each toe. The direction of pressure is from the inside to the outside, so the outside two toes are twisted toward the outside of the foot. The middle toe does not have a designated direction, so I do both directions to even things out. The inner two toes wring toward the inside of the foot. Switch the foot-holding hand in the middle of the toe-massage progression so you wring the toes in a perfect balance.

Massaging each toe individually is a challenge for those first massages. Not only do the tiny toes curl into a tight fist of phalanges, but they are so small that it seems impossible to get in between to massage them. Take it slowly so no toe is missed.

9. **Palmar kneading to the sole**: Use the palm of your hand to knead the sole of the tiny foot.

10. **Effleurage**: Do three effleurages again, from toes to hip, and then finish off with reflex stroking.

Transition: I like to move from the front of leg massage to leg pumping (pages 149–151). I massage the backs of the legs after giving the back massage.

Legs (posterior)

1. **Effleurage**: Starting at the foot, wrap your hands across the leg and spread the coconut oil up the leg to the hip. Include the gluteals as you wrap around the hip and split your hands to run down either side of the leg back to the foot without pressure. The pressure of this stroke is up toward the heart and light on the way back. Do this starting effleurage stroke three times or more.

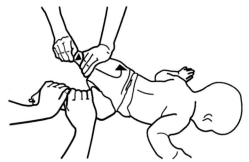

Figure 7.16. Tandem effleurage to posterior legs. If there's a diaper on, just go up and over the hip.

2. **Reinforced palmar kneading**: Bridge your effleurage with a half-effleurage up the leg and then start reinforced palmar kneading to the entire hip area, including the glutes. Place one hand on top of the other hand and do a cup-shaped (fingertips down) palmar kneading to the hip three times, including the gluteal area. When the baby has diapers on, then I work on top of the diapers. This stroke helps loosen up the hip to get the digestive system moving or for leg pumping.

3. **Fingertip and thumb kneading to the hip**: Knead the hip with alternate thumb kneading, single-handed fingertip and single-handed thumb kneading. Work the hip thoroughly before working down the back of the leg.

4. **Wringing to the upper leg**: The hamstring muscles start at the ischial tuberosity (sit bones) and go to the back of the knee, attaching to the upper part of the lower leg. Put your hands across the leg and wring along this entire length. Be sure your wringing strokes include the lower attachments.

5. **Alternate thumb kneading to the popliteal fossa (back of knee)**: The back of the knee is an intersection of attachments of the upper and lower leg. As this is a rapidly growing person with legs that are getting stronger everyday, there is a lot to do here. Wrap your fingers around the knee, pointing the fingers up toward the trunk of the body, and massage extensively from back to front with fingertip kneading, feeling for all the delicate attachments of the hamstrings and the gastrocnemius. Then use alternate thumb kneading around those same attachments.

6. **Wringing and alternate thumb kneading to the lower leg**: My bridging stroke between the upper and lower leg is usually wringing from the top of the upper leg to the bottom of the gastrocnemius and the Achilles attachment at the baby's heel. I also add in some tiny alternate thumb kneading strokes as the baby moves its leg back and forth. Just go with the flow.

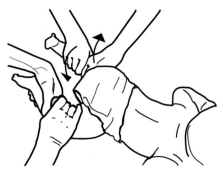
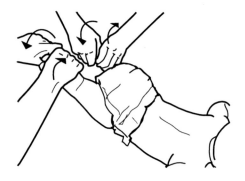

Figure 7.17. Tandem wringing massage to the leg in prone position.

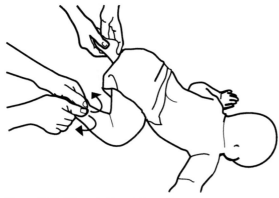

Figure 7.18. Alternate thumb kneading.

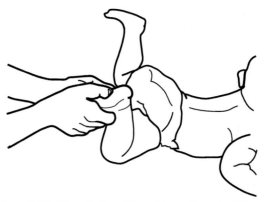

Figure 7.20. Alternate thumb kneading to the sole of the foot.

7. **Alternate thumb kneading to the foot**: With the foot flexed and the knee bent so the lower leg is pointing to the sky, massage the sole of the foot with both of your thumbs in a slow alternate thumb kneading. Bending the leg at the knee makes massaging the foot very easy and it fits into your hand well. The Babinski reflex is the movement of the big toe toward the top of the foot and a curling of the other toes. The reflex is initiated through stimulation to the foot and toes.

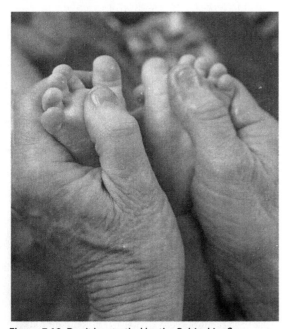

Figure 7.19. Don't be startled by the Babinski reflex. Nothing is going wrong: the reflex is perfectly natural in children up to about two years.

8. **Wringing to the sole of the foot**: I usually lean my elbows on the table or surface that we are massaging the baby on for steadiness and endurance, and I do a thumb wringing to the sole of the foot. You always will get a reflex from these stimulating massage moves.

9. **Bilateral thumb kneading to the ankle bones**: Cup the baby's heel in both hands with the thumbs moving around the ankle bones. Do this firmly and slowly with two thumbs working at the same pace on opposite ankles (simultaneous thumb kneading) and then alternate the thumbs. Alternate thumb kneading and simultaneous thumb kneading are great for loosening up all of the strong tendinous attachments to those boney structures

Digestive Massage

The baby massage that makes the most impact in the first days, weeks, and months of life is the digestive massage. Many babies experience painful gas or other digestive problems. This may cause them to cry frequently and inconsolably, in a condition commonly known as "colic." Not all excessive crying is caused by digestive problems, but it's certainly worth trying massage if your baby appears "colicky" or is having obvious digestive problems. I have always used a combination of massage and leg pumping as my best remedy for even the toughest digestive problems.

The problems of constipation and indigestion for babies can be due to an inherited predisposition or to the mother's postpartum eating habits. Some babies seem sluggish from the very beginning of their digestive career, while others are the opposite, with food flying through them. Whether the peristaltic action of the digestive system is too fast or too slow, the massage for the digestive tract is the same. Most strokes are pretty straightforward and should be familiar to you from doing the pregnancy massages.

1. **Effleurage**: I usually start with effleurage on the front to accustom the baby to my touch and to give me a chance to collect some tactile

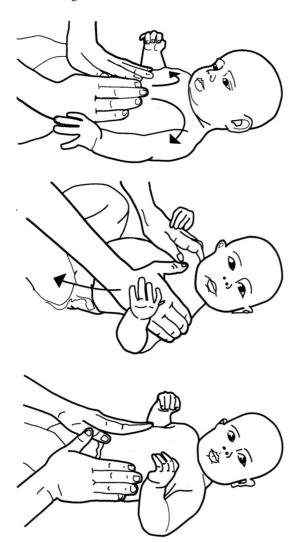

Figure 7.21. Baby anterior effleurage.

information as I travel around the front of the trunk from the lower to upper areas of the tummy and chest.

Effleurage can be done from the front, face-to-face, going up and out to the shoulders and around to the back of the shoulder and then down the sides and looping around to start up the tummy and chest again. It can also be done standing at the head of the baby, going down the chest and tummy with the whole palmar surface, around to the sides, and then pulling up the sides to the armpits and around the shoulders and then up into the back of the neck. Do this three times, starting again in the front with your hands on the upper chest.

The point is to do an all-encompassing stroke that covers the entire front of the baby and gets up and around the shoulders and travels down the sides, whether aiming with an upward or a downward stroke.

2. **Palmar kneading**: Continue your effleurage, but mix in some gentle overhanded palmar kneading to the abdomen, which may be distended. With increasing pressure, move in a clockwise direction around the abdomen, starting at the lower right hand side. For babies one month and under, start with light abdominal massage and gradually increase pressure. In general, don't massage the abdomen just after the baby has eaten.

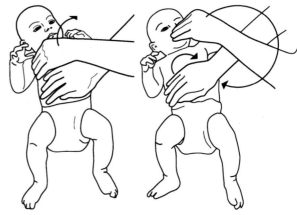

Figure 7.22. Overhanded palmar kneading to the abdomen.

THE PROBLEM OF PROJECTILE VOMITING

If your baby suffers from projectile vomiting, you will want to massage before, during, and after eating. Your massage will be trying to re-pattern the baby by changing tension patterns with touch and scrambling the signals for vomiting. Try some gentle open C-shaped scooping to the front of the baby's neck. Massaging the throat helps to disturb the buildup of tension that produces projectile vomiting.

3. **Wringing**: Follow kneading with wringing by placing your hands side by side, pulling and pushing opposite each other across the entire abdomen, wrapping right around to the back. I do these criss-cross strokes about ten times, gently at the beginning and then more firmly to ease up general tension in the tummy.

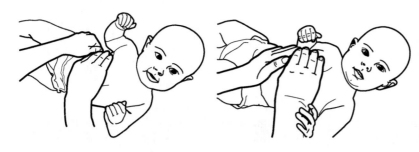

Figure 7.23. Unilateral wringing. You might want to move from bilateral to unilateral wringing and then back to bilateral.

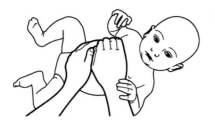
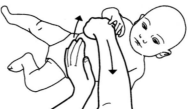
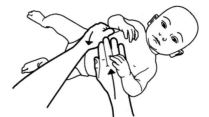

Figure 7.24. Bilateral wringing.

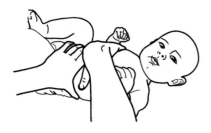

Figure 7.25. You can also do your wringing with an open C-shape to your hand.

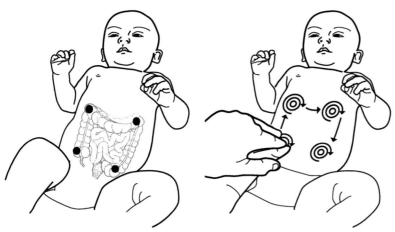

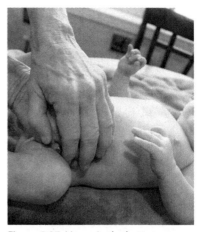

Figure 7.26. Fingertip kneading around the digestive tract.

Figure 7.27. Linger in the bottom corner of the digestive tract to help clear up constipation.

4. **Fingertip kneading**: Now use reinforced fingertip kneading and single-handed fingertip kneading for the square shape of the large intestine's path around the abdomen. Stack your hands one on top of the other and keep the fingers straight and stiff so the fingertips are very focused and do not take up a lot of skin space on the baby's abdomen. Then knead with a pivoting action of your wrist so the fingertips are like a soft-tipped drill. Start at the lower aspect of the abdomen on the baby's right-hand side where the small intestine hooks up to the large intestine. In this corner, make a slow start by massaging in one place for a while. Work your way up the ascending colon to the first corner (flexure), where it turns just under the costal angle of the tiny ribs.

Stop there and linger again before heading across the abdomen (the transverse colon). Pause in the upper left corner. This is usually where all the trouble starts, where the colon not only turns a corner, but also starts to change body level from front to back. This part of the digestive tract is a natural slow-down place. It can be a really problematic intersection with impacted contents, so give it lots of attention before starting your massage down the descending colon. Also linger in the lower left corner for a few minutes.

5. **Vibrations**: The vibration massage stroke is like getting "nervous." You can do this fine shaking stroke with all sorts of different parts of your hand. The most common is the palmar whole-handed vibration. This stroke is stationary. Place your hands in one place on the baby's tummy and vibrate as finely as you can. I stand so my hands are across the baby's abdomen. I put my two hands next to each other and they seem to help each other out!

This first palmar vibration is followed by a reinforced palmar vibration making sure that the tips of the fingers are curved downward and not lifting up. Using the entire palmar surface including the fingers, you can move this reinforced palmar vibration around the baby's abdomen, no matter how small it is. Sustain these vibrations for about a minute at a time. You can also do static reinforced fingertip vibrations and running fingertip vibrations. Your hands might move side to side or up and down—use whatever method gives you the finest vibration.

Work from the lower left side in a counter-clockwise direction, or start at the junction of the small and large intestine in the lower right-hand side of the baby, right where the hip bone is, and into the softness of the lower corner of the abdomen.

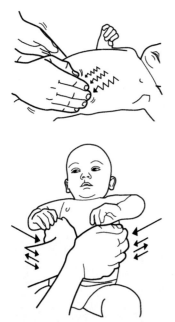

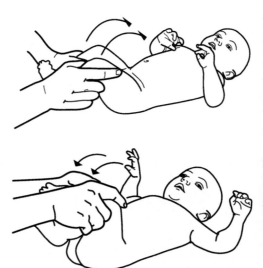

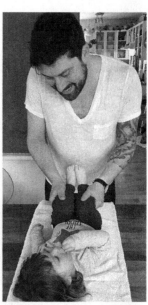

Figure 7.28. Vibrations can go side to side or up and down.

Figure 7.29. Simultaneous leg pumping.

Figure 7.30. Jeremy and Frances demonstrate simultaneous leg pumping.

I tend to use the palmar vibration starting with the baby on its side and sandwiched between my hands, one hand on the back and one hand on the tummy. I vibrate my palms in one spot, followed by the running vibrations to ascending, transverse and descending colons. I go in one direction and also in the other. Either way you are safe; nothing can go wrong. The tummy will untangle with the strokes, exciting a slow colon and slowing down a fast-tracking colon. With your focused attention to the large intestine, you will help to "normalize" the tummy problems, if any.

Focus on the lower digestive tract (end of the colon) to leave it open, relaxed, and hopefully more responsive. The baby will usually pee by now as massage relaxes the sphincters and the let-down reflexes will respond. Little boy babies are like firehoses, so get extra protection for your massage surface. Even with protection, I still get sprayed on a regular basis. It is what I call a positive problem.

6. **Leg pumping**: Leg pumping is the best approach for unwinding the digestive system. It is like taking a walk around the block.

When we mobilize the hips, the baby's entire digestive system is stimulated, giving a peristaltic action to the contents of the large intestine. There are three kinds of leg pumping to include before, during, and after the tummy rub.

- **Simultaneous leg pumping**: Bend the baby's legs in to the tummy gently and firmly. This is done by holding the baby's leg at the ankles and waiting for an opening in the baby's leg movements. Babies with digestive problems tend to hold their legs stiff, straight, and stretched out in front of them, or sometimes they tuck their legs tightly to their tummy with the same symptoms. In either situation, wait for an opening to move and bend the legs in and out.

I hold the legs with a finger under the back of each knee to encourage the baby to let go of the tension in the knee and bend. Because the hips are not fully formed and strong, be sure to keep a very straight angle to the leg. Do not angle the leg out to the side; keep it in a straight line as it flexes toward the abdomen.

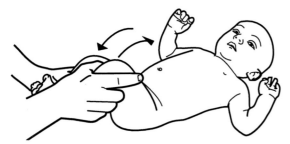
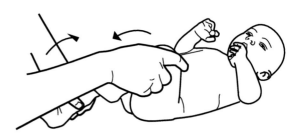

Figure 7.31. Alternate leg pumping.

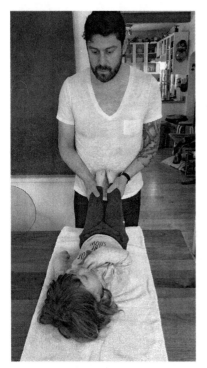
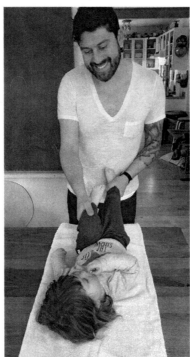
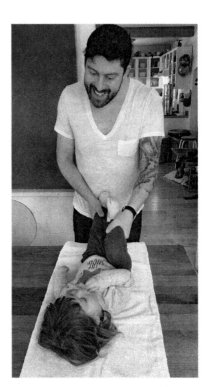

Figure 7.32. Alternate leg pumping.

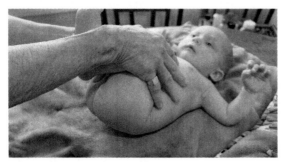
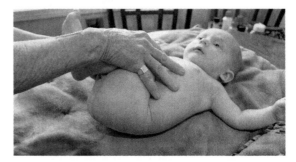

Figure 7.33. Rotational movement.

- **Alternate leg pumping**: With the same handgrip, hold the legs for a straight knee bend to the abdomen. Bend one leg and then straighten it out completely before bending the other knee. Do this at least ten times.

- **Rotational movement**: Bend both legs up to the abdomen and then wrap your hands around the legs to keep everything together in a little package. Then start to roll the whole lower body around in a circular movement, with the low back (lumbar area) getting a circular massage from the surface. This puts gentle pressure on the sacrum, which is the source of nerves for the digestive area.

Do the three kinds of leg pumping for a few minutes. I repeat this series of movements more than once at ten times each, minimum.

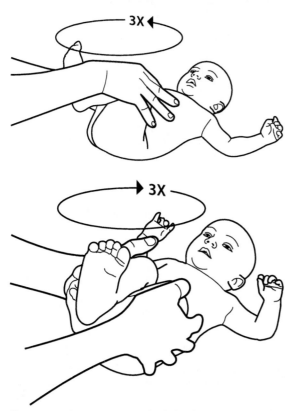

Figure 7.34. Be sure to rotate the baby three times in each direction.

This is great to do after the tummy massage and then follow it with another abdominal massage. So in summary: massage, leg pump, massage, leg pump. *Ad infinitum!*

Side-lying digestive massage

This is a cozy way to relieve a tummy ache. Put the baby on its side and hold it between your hands in a "comfort sandwich." Do circles with the whole palmar aspect of your hands, one hand on the back of the baby and the other hand on the front of the baby. Move your hands with the same speed and momentum. The abdominal hand is always going clockwise from the right-hand side over to the left and around (following the digestive tract in its natural peristaltic direction). The hand on the back of the baby follows the same speed, size of stroke, and momentum, but in a counterclockwise direction. When the front hand is at the top of the circle of the stroke, the back hand is at the bottom, and vice versa. It is like pedaling a bike, but we are pedaling a baby. This all-encompassing stroke is calming and soothing for the parents too.

To perfectly balance the baby massage, turn the baby to the other side and perform the same technique. This means you're doing alternate palmer kneading as described in the paragraph above, but with the baby flipped to the other side. This is a good starter stroke for the side-lying technique and also a good ending stroke.

In the middle, do some focused abdominal massage work using your fingertips. With one hand supporting the back, use the other hand to

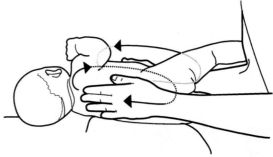

Figure 7.35. For side-lying digestive massage, rotate the hand on the abdomen in one direction and the hand on the back in the other.

work into the tummy with some single-handed fingertip kneading. Move in the direction of the digestive system (up the right side of the tummy, across, down the left side, and across to the start), remembering to linger in the corners.

After massaging the baby's digestive system directly from the front, work indirectly on the baby's back. Use single-handed fingertip kneading along the back muscles, particularly the erector spinae that stretch from the base of the skull to the sacrum. Fingertip kneading along those back muscles can soothe cramping in the abdominal area by working out tension in the low back.

Finishing strokes for digestive massage

Do effleurage and light reflex stroking to finish off this massage. The light reflex stroking can be mesmerizing and soothing, helping to anesthetize the area of discomfort without any pressure, just light sensation to override the tension and cramping pain underneath the surface of the skin.

I do the light reflex stroking the same way I do the overhanded palmar kneading, where one hand chases the other hand around the baby's tummy in the direction of the digestive flow, up the right-hand side of the baby's tummy and down the left-hand side. I also do light reflex stroking back and forth in a modified wringing. You can also use the back of your hand for this wringing. The back of the hand, including the fingers, is so soft compared to the palmar surface that it is a good way to finish.

Respiratory Baby Massage

Respiratory problems in babies are treated in much the same way as respiratory problems in adults. Many issues result from cold or flu, the same as in adults. Some infant complaints can result from complications of the delivery. Others have a genetic origin. However, no matter what the cause, simple massage techniques can help the baby breathe easier and help the parents relax!

Treating chest congestion

Problems with the respiratory system often involve lung congestion. Generally speaking, the basic approach to treating chest congestion is to loosen up phlegm in the lungs with basic massage strokes for the chest and thoracic area and then use specific respiratory massage strokes such as rib raking, percussion (cupping), and compression. This massage will make coughing more productive because the phlegm causing congestion is loosened up and can be expelled from the body.

Certain postures can also help the baby expel phlegm. Many of these postures can also be used to treat an adult with a respiratory problem.

1. **Effleurage and palmar kneading to the anterior trunk**: Spend a couple minutes spreading the oil over the front of the baby, followed by palmer kneading to the chest and shoulders.

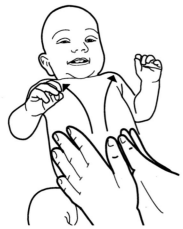

Figure 7.36. Spread oil with an easy effleurage.

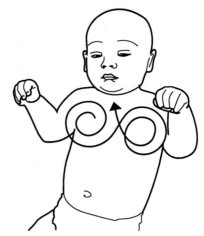

Figure 7.37. Palmar kneading to the chest and shoulders. Be sure to wrap right around the shoulders.

2. **Costal-angle stroking**: Face-to-face with the baby, put both thumbs together in the middle of the bottom of the baby's sternum, where you will find the xiphoid process, that little projection of soft bone just below the central apex of the arch of the ribs, where they meet in the middle. Place your thumbs together at the top point of the costal angle.

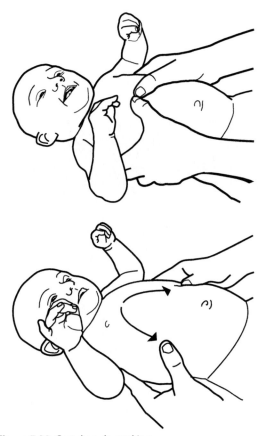

Figure 7.38. Costal-angle stroking.

Then slide your hands evenly and slowly down the opposite sides of the ribs, letting your thumbs slide underneath the edge of the ribs. This movement stretches the diaphragm muscle that attaches along this border. This stroking has pressure on the downward stroke and no pressure coming back up—lift your hands when returning to the xiphoid process. Slowly is the key for the downward stroke. Do the costal-angle stroking at least ten times.

3. **Rib raking**: This stroke stretches the little muscles between the ribs and immediately provides needed elasticity to make baby's breathing easier. Standing at the side of the baby (I swivel the baby on the towel, turning the whole towel or mat instead of picking up the baby), use a claw-like grip with your fingertips as though you are playing the piano. Place both hands underneath the baby, with your fingertips (be right on the tips of your fingers) in between the ribs. Pull up toward you, stretching the tiny intercostal muscles. Do this movement three or four times slowly.

Now use one hand at a time to rake the ribs on the side of the baby's body farthest from you. This is an overhanded rib raking in which one hand starts the stroke just as the other hand is finishing. Once you've raked the ribs about ten times on one side, swivel the towel to do the other side. I sometimes go from one side to the other twice. Sometimes I do another round of costal-angle stoking between switching sides for rib raking.

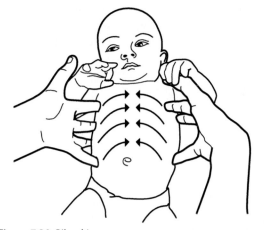

Figure 7.39. Rib raking.

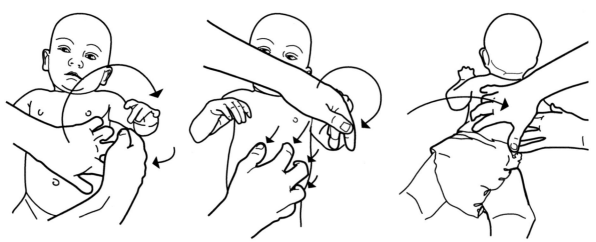

Figure 7.40. Overhanded rib raking.　　　　　　**Figure 7.41.** Posterior rib raking.

4. **Palmar kneading to the shoulders**: This is a general stroke to stimulate circulation throughout the baby's chest. Face-to-face with the baby, knead in a figure-eight pattern around the shoulders and across the chest with your palms. This stretches and stimulates the pectoral muscles that are important for respiratory function. The figure eight will help you keep the direction of pressure up and away from the center.

5. **Reinforced palmar kneading to the chest**: With one hand on top of the other in a stack, and with the direction of pressure always up and out from the center, from the sternum out toward the shoulders, again stretch the pectoral muscles, a focal point in the respiratory treatment.

6. **Tapotement and postural drainage**: Cupping will help loosen up any mucus or other unwanted fluid in the lungs. Use cupping all over the trunk of the body. Support the baby with one hand on the tummy in side-lying. Hook its leg over your supportive hand. Shape your other hand as though you are scooping water out of a creek and gently thump the entire back from the lumbar area upwards to over the shoulders. This stroke is the same as the kind of tapping you'd use to burb a baby after nursing. In fact, you can do this stroke with the baby held against you as you continue

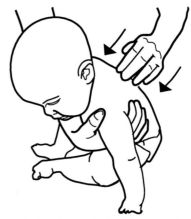

Figure 7.42. Cupping to the back in a seated position.

the cupping tapotement and move your body up and down.

The only place not to use cupping is directly on the spine itself.

Although the back is tiny, there is still room for this stimulating stroke to activate coughing and clearing of the breathing passageways. Rub the back with firm one-handed effleurages before and after the application of cupping. Although cupping is stimulating at first, if it continues for some time, it then has the opposite effect of calming and anesthetizing the area.

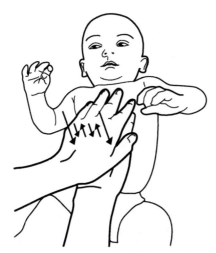

Figure 7.43. Thoracic compression. This gentle pumping is designed to help clear the lungs. I often use a compression stroke when the baby is in the inverted posture on my lap, head down, as well as on the horizontal, as seen here. I'll do compressions about three times and then return to a round of massage strokes, then more compressions, and then more massage. These can be life-saving strokes to clear the lungs.

This stroke is important to keep in your daily baby massage skill set. You want your baby to be accustomed to the full repertoire of strokes in case your little one is in distress and you need to have some remedies at your fingertips in the middle of the night.

Perform each drainage position with full body jostling, shaking, and bouncing. Just bounce your body or leg with the baby bouncing on it.

- **Upper lobe drainage**: Place the baby on your lap so it's in a seated position. This position will drain the upper lobe.
- **Middle lobe drainage**: Place the baby in side-lying across your knees.
- **Lower lobe drainage**: Lay the baby on your lap with its head toward your knees. Lower your knees so the baby is inverted with its head lower than its body.

In general, side-lying position is one of the easiest ways to get the lungs activated and is a good drainage position for respiratory

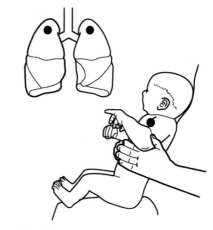

a. Upper lobe drainage position

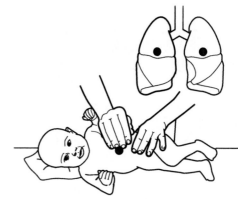

b. Side-lying middle lobe drainage position

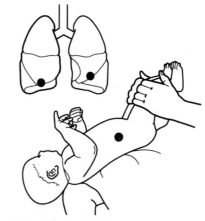

c. Lower lobe drainage position

Figure 7.44. Drainage positions for the lungs. Once the mucus is loosened, a variety of postures can help drain phlegm from the lungs.

congestion. Use lots of finishing effleurages and light reflex stroking to complete the sequence.

7. **Light reflex stroking**: This is important to include, especially over surfaces where you might have used compression or some other uncomfortable respiratory moves like cupping. The finale of light reflex stroking for your respiratory baby massage is like an eraser that ensures the baby will not remember any tactile discomfort, although it might have saved its life.

I use two or three styles of light reflex stroking:

- Simultaneous stroking with the tips of the fingers.
- Intermittent light fingertip tapping on the length of the thoracic area.
- Light caressing with the backs of my fingers.

I also do a featherweight wringing across the back, arms, legs, abdomen, and chest. Although such skin stimulation wakes up the nervous system, in the long run it has a soothing effect. I learned this technique from parents of special-needs kids, such as those with cerebral palsy or muscular dystrophy. They invented this type of wringing and many other playful strokes to provide neurological stimulation for their kids.

Sinus massage

The respiratory system also includes the ear, nose, and throat, which can also be drained through massage. Begin by giving the baby a basic head massage. You can use the same strokes as in the adult massage (see page 52). Then focus on the sides of the nose where it attaches to the face.

1. **Running nasal shaking**: Make a C-shape with the hand, with the pointer finger and the thumb making contact along the border of the nose where it attaches to the face. Move your fingertips back and forth from side to side in a fast, but gentle fluttering motion. Run the stroke up and down the nose from the base to the top between the eyes.

2. **Nasal root shaking**: Do some gentle shaking at the bottom of the nose where it attaches to the face at the flare of the nostrils. Be careful not to pinch inward: maintain the flare entrance opening throughout the stroke.

3. **Static nasal shaking**: Perform the same shaking technique in about four locations from the bottom of the nose (the root) upwards toward the top of the nose between the eyes, shaking the sides of the nose where it attaches to the face.

4. **Nasal pressure points**: Place your thumb and pointer finger at the base of the nose at the outer flare of the nostrils like you are going to pinch the nostrils together. But instead of pinching, gently press into the face and hold it for a breath (an adult breath). Then move up to the next level and hold the pressure for another breath. Continue for about four levels of pressure, ending at the top of the nose.

5. **Running nasal shaking**: Move with gentle yet fast back and forth movements from the bottom of the nose to the top and then reverse and go back down the nose from the top to the bottom. This is a light, yet effective stroke, especially as a finishing touch for opening up the breathing through the nose.

6. **Orbital sinus stroking**:
   - **Lower edge of the eye (the infraorbital ridge)**: Place your thumbs on either side of the nose in the center of the face and trace the lower edge of the eye from the nose out to the temples. You may feel a little notch in the middle of the lower orbital ridge—this is where the sinus drainage is located.
   - **Upper edge of the eye (the supraorbital ridge)**: Place both thumbs at the center of the face on either side of the nose and trace the eyebrows out to the temples with firm pressure.

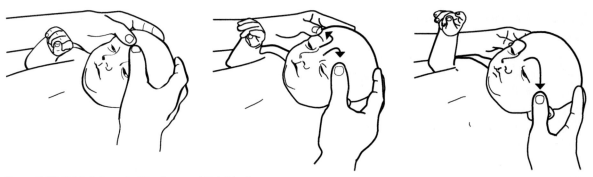

Figure 7.45. Orbital sinus stroking (supraorbital ridge).

7. **Temporal fingertip kneading**: With your fingertips squeezed together, massage around the temples along the hairline for a few minutes. Your baby may seem agitated when these sensitive areas are massaged, but persevere.

8. **Fingertip kneading**: Do some fingertip kneading around the ear where it attaches to the side of the head. This will help open up the main drainage canal, the Eustachian tube, so fluids can drain away.

9. **Passive ear rotations**: With continuous traction, pull out gently but firmly on the ears. Rotate the ear three times in one direction and three times in the other direction. You can do both ears at the same time.

10. **Light reflex stroking**: Use light reflex stroking on the face over the sinuses and from the center out toward the ears. Use both the backs of your fingers and the palmar surface of your fingers. This will encourage the flow of congested upper respiratory circulation toward the ears and Eustachian tube for drainage.

In times of respiratory trouble, do a sinus-clearing massage three times a day before breastfeeding to create a positive reward at the end of the massage. The sinus area can be sensitive, so go easy at first. As the baby gets accustomed to the sinus work, do more work on the supraorbital and infraorbital ridges.

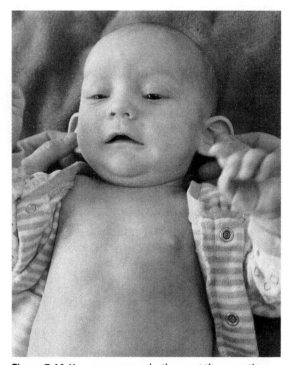

Figure 7.46. You can massage both ears at the same time.

In 1954, my friend Joni's son was born with blocked tear ducts. His eyes ran continuously, like he was crying. The doctor showed her how to do this massage, and after six months of dedicated home treatment before nursing and during bathtime, his ducts cleared.

Special Remedial Extremity Massage

Babies' overall malleability allows them to be delivered through the narrow birth canal. They are able to mold to the mom's shape, especially if they have a long, slow birth, taking the time to make their heads into a cone shape.

However, sometimes babies are delivered with injuries to shoulders that can range from dislocation to strains and sprains. After a breech birth, many babies arrive with a shoulder separation. Usually one shoulder is acutely involved with other affected, but not so severely. Massaging around the shoulders helps speed up the recovery and prevent scar tissue from forming.

Sometimes babies arrive with a partial paralysis of the arm. This is often the result of a problem in the neck, sometimes due to the turning of the neck by a hurried helper as part of a life-saving measure. No matter what the reason, I get to work massaging as soon as I can to get that injury healing faster, first helping to dissipate any inflammatory signs and symptoms and then to help build good blood circulation in the area so the arm is not "jammed" with the natural immobility of the paralysis.

Putting parents to work on these problems is very rewarding. It helps them feel less helpless and they can affect change immediately.

Infantile torticollis

Infantile torticollis, or wry neck, happens when babies are in the womb in an upright position for weeks. Their head tilts to the side, resulting in a kink in the neck when they are born. The sooner the baby starts massage therapy, the faster its twisted neck can be remedied. This condition always involves the sternocleidomastoid (SCM) muscle in the front and on the sides of the neck. This muscle helps to move the head from side-to-side and to rotate the face. In torticollis, one side of the neck has overly contracted muscles while the other side is overly stretched.

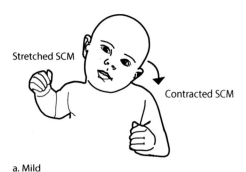

a. Mild

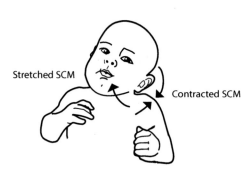

In severe cases, the head is pulled into rotation toward the stretched side.

b. Severe

Figure 7.47. Infantile torticollis (wry neck).

Although it sounds extreme, I have treated newborns with the SCM muscle in the side of the neck folded right over. In extreme cases, the condition requires surgery. One mom I worked with massaged her baby diligently and was successful in avoiding an operation for his severe torticollis.

This treatment is very straightforward, with two principles at work. One is to loosen the contracted muscle and the other is to strengthen the muscle on the weak side. This treatment for torticollis can also be used for babies with a slight deviation in the angle of the head. Although I have only treated about a dozen cases of official torticollis in my practice, I've had many babies that have a favored side and slight neck or head tilt problem.

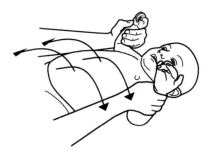

a. Roll the baby side to side to gain general mobility in the head, neck, and shoulders. The baby will naturally use its SCM muscles to resist the rolling movements.

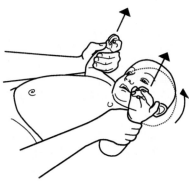

b. Supine trunk flexion to encourage bilateral strengthening of the neck muscles. Lift the baby straight up. The baby will use its SCM to lift its head.

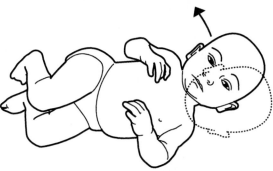

c. Side-lying with the contracted side down will strengthen the stretched side of the SCM as the baby lifts its head.

Figure 7.48. Exercises to strengthen the neck muscles bilaterally. All three movements elicit the baby's natural reflex of lifting its head. This movement against gravity strengthens the SCM muscles.

THREE EXERCISES TO STRENGTHEN A STRETCHED SCM

Hold the baby firmly on its side on a horizontal surface such as your lap. Support the body with both hands so the baby is comfortable and secure. One hand should be under the baby, cupping its head on the side with the contracted muscle.

a. **Little lifts**: Lift the baby's head a few inches and relax your hands. Repeat three times. Rest and massage in between with fingertip kneading on the contracted side and light reflex stroking on both sides.

b. **Bounce the baby's head with larger lifts**: At the same time, raise the baby toward a more upright position, so the baby's neck works harder to lift its head. Massage in between.

c. **Tilting downwards**: Tilt the baby's body downward by laying it on your thighs and slowly letting your feet slide out. You can

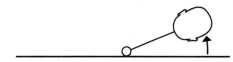

a. Side-lying lift

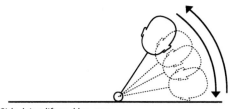

b. Side-lying lift and bounce

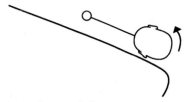

c. Lifting from a downward tilt

Figure 7.49. Side-lying exercises to strengthen the stretched SCM as the baby works to lift its head.

bounce your knees gently, but the main idea is again to encourage the natural flexing reflexes as the baby lifts its head against gravity. Again, massage in between.

Always end the exercises with massage and light reflex stroking to the neck. Massaging with a light touch will erase the muscle memory if the exercises were uncomfortable.

UNILATERAL SCM FLEXION WITH FACE ROTATION TO THE CONTRACTED (SHORTENED) SIDE

Stabilize the baby's shoulder with your hand as you do the following movements. You want to prevent the baby's shoulder from following the head as you move it.

- **For mild torticollis**: Hold the baby's head at the back slightly to the top of the head. Flex the baby's ear to shoulder on the stretched side while stabilizing the shoulder on the other side of the baby's body. (Figure 7.50)

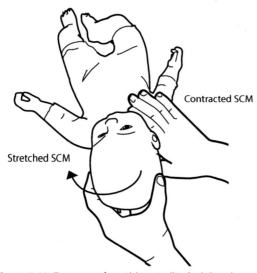

Figure 7.50. Treatment for mild torticollis. Stabilize the baby's shoulder on the contracted side, and move the baby's ear gently towards its shoulder on the other side, stretching the contracted side of the baby's neck.

With severe torticollis, you can often use two people—one to stabilize the shoulders and one to flex and rotate the head. You want to flex toward the stretched side with the face rotating toward the contracted side. (Figure 7.51)

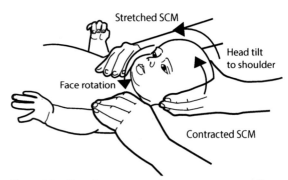

Figure 7.51. If you have two people, one person can stabilize the shoulders and the other can tilt and rotate the head.

- **For severe torticollis**: Hold the shoulder down on the contracted side and apply slight compression. Use the other hand to tilt the baby's ear to the shoulder on the stretched side. At the same time, rotate the baby's head toward the contracted side. Massage in between.
- **For severe torticollis**: Hold the baby's head at the back, secure at the neck. Gently move the ear to shoulder on the stretched side and rotate the face toward the contracted side. (Figures 7.52 and 7.53) Massage in between to soften the adhesions and lengthen the contracted SCM.

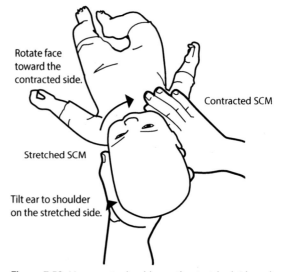

Figure 7.52. Move ear to shoulder on the stretched side and rotate the head toward the contracted side. This is a tricky movement to master, so try it on a doll first! The movement puts the baby into a mirror image of its torticollis (severe).

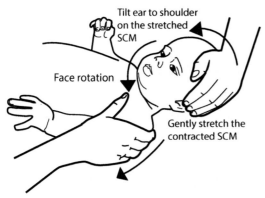

Figure 7.53. Another option for this movement, but with a face-to-face position.

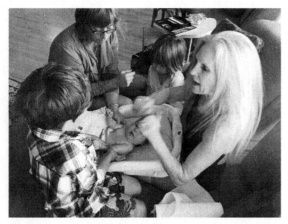

Figure 7.54. Friends of all ages and genders can be taught to help with baby massage, especially remedial treatments like this one for infant torticollis. The more massages, the faster the recovery.

Teething

The symptoms of a teething baby—restlessness, indigestion, and fussiness—can be treated with a general full-body massage. You can also use your fingertips to gently massage the jaw area and temples while the baby is contently breastfeeding.

Massaging along the gums of the baby with your fingers can also be effective. I recommend cooling your fingers in an ice bath (cold water with ice cubes in a bowl) to massage above the gum line, along the inside of the jaw, and along the gum line itself. Parents instinctively run their fingers along the baby's gums to identify where the next tooth will appear. Usually the baby's unhappy mood is

a direct correlation to a new tooth being ready to break through. A cold finger massage along the gum line will help soothe the local inflammatory response created before a new tooth pops. This is the same idea as using frozen soothers for these trying teething times.

Weaning

Massage can also help weaning children. Whether a child is nine months or three years, massage to positively reinforce the experience of being without the breast. Provide massage on the breastfeeding timetable. Massage especially at night and before or after bath time to ensure a deeper sleep and provide a repatterning experience.

Massage is a good way for the mom to maintain intimacy and experience loving contact while weaning from breastfeeding. She will sleep better knowing that she has given the best breast replacement with the power of her touch. The non-nursing parent is included on the weaning massage team too, of course!

Fussiness

Happy babies are easy baby-massage scenarios. Some babies are calm and quiet for the entire full-body massage, including the respiratory, digestive, and neurological massage techniques. But those babies are rare. Most babies show a predictable pattern: they get fussy and then conk out!

A relaxed baby is not always a quiet baby. When babies are thoroughly massaged, they are affected in a comprehensive and protracted way. The initial behavior can typically be cooing and chewing. This may evolve into a fussiness that indicates apparent fatigue, signaling that we are having an effect on the entire system. The fussiness is not a negative outcome but rather a reaction to overall full-body stimulation. It is a natural discharge of the input of electric-like currents that are felt throughout the baby's body.

Fussiness is naturally interpreted by first-time baby massagers as the time to quit. The assume that the fussiness is how the baby is saying "Stop."

However, the fussing is actually an indication of the short-term effects of the massage. The massage experience is typically one of letting go of tension and then falling into sleep and/or deep relaxation. When babies are going to fall asleep, they often become noisy or fussy.

So persist and complete your full-body massage. Expect a fussy baby, but don't assume that means something is wrong. Simply put, your baby is unwinding with sound effects.

"I enjoyed the first baby massage. It was a chance for me to bond with Inara, and I hoped that she'd be able to sense that I was trying to make her feel better. She didn't seem overly impressed with the effort though! Now, I usually lightly massage her during bathtime—she's less squirmy than when she's out of the tub. I think she enjoys the physical interaction, and I think it's really good for my relationship with her. It's a good opportunity to bond with my baby, and it's a good way for me to bond with Fallon [Inara's mom] when we get to share these moments." —Darren

---

The baby may need to fuss through that initial cycle of stimulation to reach the secondary effect of deeper relaxation. If you don't keep massaging through the noisy fussiness, you may never acquire the longer-term benefits of your baby massages.

If you massage every day, you will learn different responses from your baby, who may give you good baby-massage days and challenging baby-massage days. Your baby may also respond differently at different times of the day to the same massage. As the baby grows and changes physically, the massages change and the baby's reactions change too.

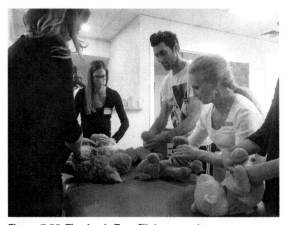

Figure 7.55. The Apple Tree Clinic maternity massage workshop uses newborn-infant-sized teddy bears for future parents to try out leg massage and leg pumping. All massage strokes and postural drainage positions are easily practiced to give the parents some hands-on massage practice that will be needed when the baby arrives.

Taking It to the Streets

My goal is to deliver the hands-on skills needed for massage anywhere and everywhere babies are being born. Hopefully this will change the world for the better, one massage at a time. My lifelong passion for social activism stems from the social, political, and educational changes in society I witnessed in the sixties and seventies. In my teens, the teachings of Socrates influenced my thinking about education and the value of gatherings and the power of passing along an idea that just gets better as it is passed from person to person. Education remains, for me, that spark that ignites between like-minded people.

In my first career, I was an audiovisual specialist. Like others at the time, I was influenced by Marshall McLuhan's 1967 message that *the medium is the message*—that we can communicate intensely and intimately with each other through evolving social media. In those days, for me this meant running five slide projectors at one time and having multimedia educational "happenings." I was able to use his disruption of conventional reporting and give people a more experiential way of learning.

I became intrigued with the ways we can communicate using technology and touch, two widely diverse mediums. Now, years later, his influence stays with me, but now "the medium is the *massage*," helping me integrate my two careers. I can share what I know to places I cannot physically go in the fastest way possible using Skype, FaceTime, and other communications technology.

Experiential education—old-fashioned hands-on mentoring, shoulder-to-shoulder learning, side-by-side apprenticing with more experienced practitioners—has always been my way of learning best. Two men, in particular, mentored my beginnings in massage: gestalt therapist Brian Carpendale and chaplain Don Grayston.

I was blessed to be under the influence of Brian Carpendale, who trained firsthand with Fritz Perls, the fellow who created gestalt therapy and brought psychotherapy into a more experiential medium of encounter groups and retreats. It was Brian who suggested that I expand my love of hands-on animal husbandry to include people and attend a professional massage training program.

Don Grayston was the chaplain at Selkirk College, where I was on his chaplaincy committee. Don took me to a conference where I had my first professional massage, a massage that changed my life forever. Don also gave me my first teaching job in his training program for marriage enrichment counsellors at the Anglican Synod of Canada. To the day they died, both Don and Brian were at the tips of my fingers in their last moments. It was a time of giving back what I had been so richly given: the gift of touch, the miracle of renewal.

Don and Brian, plus the work of Marshall McLuhan, gave me support to transplant the skin-on-skin ideas of Ashley Montagu and make touching a powerful gift of social activism in my life. This was the integration of my professional and personal ambitions: the desire to teach families around the world to give each other the gift of touch. The medium of massage is my transportation vehicle for passing the power of touch into the hands of children who will change the world for the better.

The true activism of holistic maternity massage starts at home, with our families, from grandparents to grandchildren. I want to change the world of tactility within families. I want to teach siblings to massage their pregnant moms and then their newborn brothers and sisters. Stories of my families who have integrated massage over the past twenty to forty years have inspired me to take this message to the streets.

Doing massage at home on a daily basis will create a ripple effect. Throughout that child's life, massage will keep the power of touch positively affecting change. We will create a future of educated touch. Kids like my daughter Crystal, who are massaged from the beginning and who have seen movies of their first massages, continue the family tradition with their own babies. Each day, Crystal massages her daughter; I hope the tradition of massage will continue with the next generation. I am counting on this.

Years ago, I had a single mother patient who had triplets through the help of medical technology. This Nelson family still uses all the massage techniques I taught the mother through her pregnancy, postpartum, and baby massages. The whole family is today passionate about the significance of massage and its therapeutic benefits.

Most recently, I have been delighted to help with the aches and pains of two in vitro children here in Nelson. They are now teenagers in high school promoting massage for not only their sports injuries, but also to help massage their grandparents. Again, their mother was adamant that massage help her maternity successes and disappointments. I was able to help right through her pregnancy to her successful births, including baby massage for those two boys.

Life's arrivals (births) and departures (deaths) both benefit from massage in similar ways. Our children can learn to massage their grandparents the same way they were massaged by their grandparents when they were babies and toddlers. These kids grow up to be hands-on teens, hugging in the hallways of our schools and taking their hands-on help to hospitals and long-term-care facilities. Bridging that generation gap with touch is a skill set that now needs to be brought out of hiding.

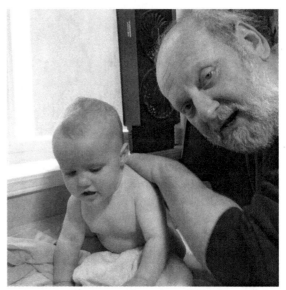

Figure 8.1. This granddad learned massage with this baby's mother, his daughter. This is second-generation baby massage! Grandfathers are hands-on now more than ever before, making their own baby massage territory.

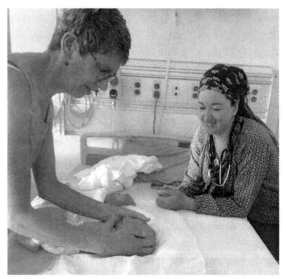

Figure 8.2. This grandmother is learning baby massage in the first hours of her granddaughter's life as the midwife looks on.

We need to take educated and appropriate touch to daycares for afternoon naps and to schools for outreach in the community massaging seniors, nurses, hospital laundry workers, teachers, and mothers for Mother's Day. We need to take these massages to the shoulders of our grandparents, saying thank you with our touch.

Despite McLuhan's warnings about our senses becoming changed and massaged by our technologies, I intend to use technology to the advantage of my cause. Spreading the message of hands-on healing through massage therapy and the extraordinary power of touch is enhanced and made easier by YouTube and Vimeo. I can teach more people with "distant demos" on YouTube than I would ever be able to "teach live" in my lifetime.

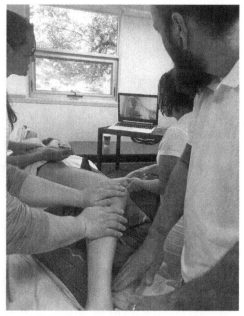

Figure 8.3. Here we're teaching Erin's mom in Nova Scotia to do the side-lying maternity massage via Skype for her training to be hands-on with her daughter's delivery in one month in British Columbia.

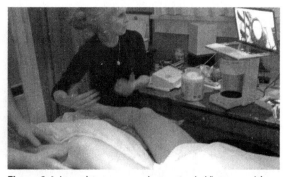

Figure 8.4. I taught a massage instructor in Vietnam with weekly classes from my clinic in Nelson.

Social Media

Social media devices may be overused in our baby deliveries in North America, but those hands that are texting just need more important skills to keep them busy.

Swapping social media for massage is a worthwhile trade, I guarantee it. With massage, skin is our medium of communication. We can show our love and affection, our support and encouragement, by massaging away those between-contraction aches and pains. We can wipe away the after-effects of each productive uterine squeeze using our hands to ease the tension.

Underlying people's need to share their secrets on social media shows our need to connect with each other on an intimate level. One person alone typing on a computer can still experience that feeling of intimacy, of one-to-one communication. The basic need for intimacy has never gone away. Yet sometimes we look in the wrong places for touch and touching to be satisfied.

Counterfeit Touch

Today, the value of touch in society is declining as inappropriate sexual touch drives out the good touch of genuine intimacy. The false currency of counterfeit touch is focused exclusively on eroticism. This is seen everywhere today in all kinds of media.

We need to restore trust in our ability to authentically touch one another. I think this would change the statistics of everything from unwanted pregnancy and unhealed sexual abuse to addictions of all kinds.

I want to make touch safe again. Good touch can heal families where touch has been affected by alcohol and drugs, causing lack of touch, abusive touch, inappropriate touch, or too much touch. This same power of touch can release body-guarded trauma and unwind the stored pain of years, months, weeks, or days of unshed tears.

Those unfortunate children raised where they were not allowed to show or express their feelings of love or affection, of fear or emotional pain, of loss and grief, can still experience healing with the simplest of comforting touch.

Healing Touch

Massaging rescue animals or abused animals is now a commonplace occurrence for me in my work. It seems I have come full circle since four-legged mammals got me started in the art of birthing in good hands. I remember how a little petting helped heal a nonpurring Siamese cat that was given to me when I was in massage school. My friends and I just passed the cat around from lap to lap as we discussed our anatomy homework. Each of us simply stroked the cat firmly and continuously. It was therapeutic stroking that started at the nose and continued to the tip of the tail. Within a day or two, the cat started purring, and within hours of that she started eating. She just needed a loving touch. No one else and nothing else had helped her to thrive. This cat was one of our first success stories.

When my massage school in Toronto had an outreach at a place called Streethaven, we regularly massaged women who wore five layers of clothing, carrying their protection beyond warmth. We massaged them through their coats and fabric armor, and we listened to their stories. With children and mothers and fathers, we can talk and touch, we can comfort with our words and with our touch, and we can ease the tension in our tone and touch alike.

I remember teaching a baby massage class through the Salvation Army home for unwed mothers as another community outreach program. The young moms in this program did not want to handle and touch their babies. I had to design ways to make them comfortable with the idea of helping their babies. Most had opted to bottle-feed. I was intrigued with how I could make the experience positive for them. These girls had no experience with positive touch. They did not know how to hand it out because they had never been handled the right way.

My students commented on the experience in a negative way, believing the girls should have reacted more positively. I remember my feedback in our group discussion was about looking at our work with this group of girls, some pregnant and some newly delivered, as an act of social activism. We were creating something brand new and we needed to make it fun and find a way "in." That was their homework. I remember telling them that this was the very reason we had the outreach program, to make a difference where it was most needed.

Today, I maintain that same drive to work where the need is most high. I still find that level of need a rewarding place to work the magic of touch. I knew then and know now that I am most useful where the need is highest, in arrivals to and departures from life.

But right here at home is another opportunity of the highest need. The LGBTQ two-spirited community is full of touching opportunities for healing the past and creating a better future for couples wanting to have a family.

My first experience was with Julie and Selena and their baby, Dénali. I have massaged these two moms and their baby girl for six years. Dénali now gives massages herself, fulfilling my desire of a new generation of children not afraid to touch. We were a great team with a message to deliver, captured in a film—*Two Moms and a Baby Girl: A Love Story*—that is a tribute to all the brave LGBTQ couples who have created new family designs. They are making the road easier to travel for those following in their footsteps.

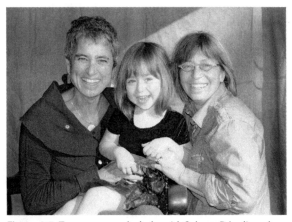

Figure 8.5. Two moms and a baby girl: Selena, Dénali, and Julie.

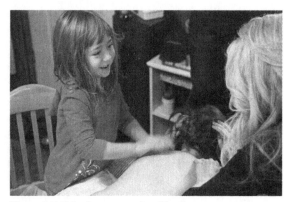

Figure 8.6. Dénali massages her friend.

More recently, I have been blessed to work with a unique couple who included me in their story as they created a family. After working with them for months, I only then found out that the rather handsome dad, complete with a trendy beard, had started out life as a female. He had transitioned and proposed to the wonderful mom, who'd already had her tubes tied when they met but agreed to reverse the process to have a child. Then, as if this wasn't all interesting enough, I found out their best man had also transitioned. He became the star of one of my pregnancy massage how-to videos; he has a special touch and way of learning I find captivating.

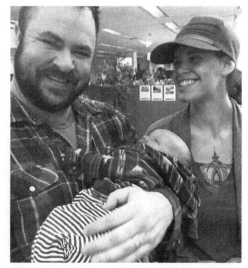

Figure 8.7. Devon and Michelle were a special delivery in every way. With Devon being transgender and Michelle having reversed her tubal ligation, Riley Francis was undoubtedly a miracle baby.

Massage was needed to help in recovery from breast removal, as well as their entire conception, pregnancy, labor, and delivery process. My work has become more expansive through special deliveries such as theirs.

Today, taking it to the streets is really taking it to our global village! Earth may be small, but electronic communication is vast. We are now more than ever before working together to create the best possible births. My global village is my dream come true, where I can teach in Vietnam every week from my laptop perched on my desk in Nelson. I work with my pregnant patient and my Vietnamese students watch and follow along, stroke by stroke and breath by breath. With technology, I've also coached a mom in Washington to massage her pregnant daughter while I worked on my own patient at home in Canada.

Ultimately, there is no limit to the possibilities for change and the power of touch. The change is right at our fingertips as it has been since the beginning of time. Each of us is here because someone had the right touch.

These tactile beginnings are also our best endings. As in pregnancy care, we also have at our fingertips the loving touch of palliative care. And for the life in between, we can now share our traditional and modern amalgamations of values to create the best world for our future and the best touch for our children. Together we can birth a better world into good hands.

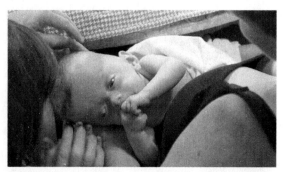

Figure 8.8. Max was born prematurely with several health concerns, including a condition called craniosynostosis, in which his skull prematurely fuses before his brain has a chance to grow. Max's family and friends will always have massage at their fingertips, showing their love and giving him their healing touch.

NOTES

Notes to Introduction

1 Bucci, R. (2017, December). "Sometimes when we touch." *BrainWorld*. Retrieved from http://brainworldmagazine.com/sometimes-when-we-touch/

2 Franklin, N. C., Mohamed, M. A., Robinson, A. T., Norkeviciute, E., & Phillips, S. A. (2014, June). "Massage therapy restores peripheral vascular function following exertion." *Archives of Physical Medicine and Rehabilitation, 95*(6): 1127–1134.

3 Keltner, D. (2010, September). "Hands on research: the science of touch." *Greater Good Magazine: Science-Based Insights for a Meaningful Life*. Retrieved from https://greatergood.berkeley.edu/article/item/hands_on_research

4 Walton, Tracy. "5 Myths and truths about massage therapy: letting go without losing heart." Massage Therapy Foundation (p. 6). Retrieved from http://www.tracywalton.com/wp-content/uploads/2016/09/5-Myths-and-Truths-about-Massage-Therapy_final-with-Page-Numers.pdf

5 Field, T. M., Schanberg, S. M., Scafidi, F., Bauer, C. R., Vega-Lahr, N., Garcia, R., Nystrom, J., & Kuhn, C. M. (1986). "Tactile/kinesthetic stimulation effects on preterm neonates." *Pediatrics, 77*(5), 654–658.

6 Field, T., Hernandez-Reif, M., Hart, S., Theakston, H., Schanberg, S., & Khun, C. (1999). "Pregnant women benefit from massage therapy." *Journal of Psychosomatic Obstetrics & Gynecology, 20*(1), 31–38.

7 Kamali, F., Panahi, F., Ebrahimi, S., & Abbasi, L. (2014). "Comparison between massage and routine physical therapy in women with sub acute and chronic nonspecific low back pain." *Journal of Back and Musculoskeletal Rehabilitation, 27*(4), 475–480.

8 Konnikova, M. (2015, March). "The power of touch." *The New Yorker*. Retrieved from https://www.newyorker.com/science/maria-konnikova/power-touch

Note to Chapter 4

9 Demirel, G. & Golbasi, Z. (2015). "Effect of perineal massage on the rate of episiotomy and perineal tearing." *International Journal of Gynecology & Obstetrics, 131*(2), 183–186.

Note to Chapter 6

10 Azriani, D., & Handayani, S. (2016). "The effect of oxytocin massage on breast milk production." *Dama International Journal of Researchers, 1*(8), 47–50.

Cho, J. S., Ahn, H. Y., Ahn, S. H., Lee, M. S., & Hur, M. H. (2012). "Effects of Oketani breast massage on breast pain, the breast milk pH of mothers, and the sucking speed of neonates." *Korean Journal of Women Health Nursing, 18*(2), 149–158.

Morhenn, V., Beavin, L. E., & Zak, P. J. (2012). "Massage increases oxytocin and reduces adrenocorticotropin hormone in humans." *Alternative Therapies in Health and Medicine, 18*(6), 11–18.

Note to Chapter 7

11 Field, T. M., Schanberg, S. M., Scafidi, F., Bauer, C. R., Vega-Lahr, N., Garcia, R., Nystrom, J., & Kuhn, C. M. (1986). "Tactile/kinesthetic stimulation effects on preterm neonates." *Pediatrics, 77*(5), 654–658.

OTHER REFERENCES

Abdallah, B., L.K. Badr, and M. Hawwari. "The efficacy of massage on short and long term outcomes in preterm infants." *Infant Behavior and Development* 36, no. 4 (Dec 2013): 662–9. https://doi.org/10.1016/j.infbeh.2013.06.009.

Ang, J.Y., J.L. Lua, A. Mathur, et al. "A randomized placebo-controlled trial of massage therapy on the immune system of preterm infants." *Pediatrics* 130, no. 6 (Dec 2012): e1549–58. https://doi.org/10.1542/peds.2012-0196.

Curties, D. *Breast Massage*. Moncton: NB: Curties-Overzet Publications Inc. 1999.

Davis, Elysia P., Laura M. Glynn, Christine Dunkel Schetter, et al. "Prenatal exposure to maternal depression and cortisol influences infant temperament." *Journal of the American Academy of Child and Adolescent Psychiatry* 46, no. 6 (2007): 737–46. https://doi.org/10.1097/chi.0b013e318047b775.

Davis, Elysia P., and Curt A. Sandman. "The timing of prenatal exposure to maternal cortisol and psychosocial stress is associated with human infant cognitive development." *Child Development* 81, no. 1 (Jan 2010): 131–48. https://doi.org/10.1111/j.1467-8624.2009.01385.x.

Diego, M.A., T. Field, and M. Hernandez-Reif. "Preterm infant weight gain is increased by massage therapy and exercise via different underlying mechanisms." *Early Human Development* 90, no. 3 (2014): 137–40. https://doi.org/10.1016/j.earlhumdev.2014.01.009.

Field, T., M. Diego, and M. Hernandez-Reif. "Preterm infant massage therapy research: a review." *Infant Behavior and Development* 33, no. 2 (Apr 2010): 115–24. https://doi.org/10.1016/j.infbeh.2009.12.004.

Fowlie, Laurel. *An Introduction to Heat & Cold as Therapy*. Toronto, ON: Curties-Overzet Publications, 2006.

Gürol, Ayşe, and Sevinç Polat. "The effects of baby massage on attachment between mothers and their infants." *Asian Nursing Research* 6, no. 1 (Mar 2012): 35–41. https://doi.org/10.1016/j.anr.2012.02.006.

Montagu, Ashley. *Touching: The Human Significance of the Skin*. Harper Collins, 1979.

Neu, M., Z. Pan, R. Workman, et al. "Benefits of massage therapy for infants with symptoms of gastroesophageal reflux disease." *Biological Research for Nursing* 16, no. 4 (Oct 2014): 387–97. https://doi.org/10.1177/1099800413516187.

Rangey, P.S., and M. Sheth. "Comparative effect of massage therapy versus kangaroo mother care on body weight and length of hospital stay in low birth weight preterm infants." *International Journal of Pediatrics* (2014): 1–4. https://doi.org/10.1155/2014/434060.

Simkin, P. *The Birth Partner: A Complete Guide to Childbirth for Dads, Doulas, and All Other Labor Companions*. 4th ed. Boston, MA: The Harvard Common Press, 2013.

Smith, S.L., S. Haley, H. Slater, et al. "Heart rate variability during caregiving and sleep after massage therapy in preterm infants." *Early Human Development* 89, no. 8 (Aug 2013): 525–9. https://doi.org/10.1016/j.earlhumdev.2013.01.004.

Tappan, F.M. *Massage Techniques: A Case Method Approach*. New York: The MacMillan Company, 1961.

Valizadeh, S., M.B. Hosseini, M. Asghari Jafarabadi, et al. "The effects of massage with coconut and sunflower oils on oxygen saturation of premature infants with respiratory distress syndrome treated with nasal continuous positive airway pressure." *Journal of Caring Sciences* 1, no. 4 (Nov 2012): 191–9.

Wang, L., J.L. He, and X.H. Zhang. "The efficacy of massage on preterm infants: a meta-analysis." *American Journal of Perinatology* 30, no. 9 (Oct 2013): 731–8. https://doi.org/10.1055/s-0032-1332801.

ONLINE CLASSROOM

Learning massage techniques is easier now with the links to the Internet. An iPad or computer can bring a massage tutorial into your bedroom in an instant. Join me in my YouTube classroom for a visual guide to many maternity massage techniques.

Baby massage

Newborn massage: https://youtu.be/7-xkO66jKhg

Baby massage: https://youtu.be/UUt4rjqVvuo

Twin baby massage:
  https://youtu.be/7-zrmH6Yxww

Teaching kids baby massage:
  https://youtu.be/N0qC8C-49oI

Two baby family massage:
  https://youtu.be/0egRbT2kMKE

Kids flash mob massage

Bridging the Gap, Fort St. John:
  https://youtu.be/OzeL0Dg7B3U

Kids and seniors: https://youtu.be/CJe9HaHhsl0

Mother's Day, Nelson: https://youtu.be/
  Z9Ey9o9HnP4

Ultimate baby massage with brothers:
  https://youtu.be/N0qC8C-49oI

Pregnancy massage

Pregnancy massage: https://www.youtube.com/
  watch?v=myvrxAsDWSA

Pregnancy massage 2: https://www.youtube.com/
  watch?v=igcNt9n5zs8

Back and head: https://youtu.be/5rP52etuX-s

Breasts (bikini top):
  https://www.youtube.com/watch?v=KHbRJ5F-
  CBTo&feature=youtu.be

Breasts (no bikini top):
  https://www.youtube.com/watch?v=2Jz-
  KL0UH7jQ&feature=youtu.be

Constipation prevention:
  https://youtu.be/QhS2y-Ox-QQ

Legs and arms: https://youtu.be/lYVwM4hrSxQ

Swollen legs: https://youtu.be/qzGNxPjhImw

Tummy, shoulders, back:
  https://youtu.be/Za7dBbzEkNM

Team massage

Massaging the team:
  https://youtu.be/eaV9dpVejcs

Vietnam maternity massage

Full maternity massage:
  https://youtu.be/20AyXhNz3YU

Teaser: https://youtu.be/kfNUeJCrq18

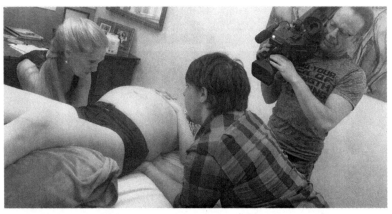

The camera shines a light on what words find difficult to describe.

ACKNOWLEDGMENTS

A heartfelt thank you to the following:

Midwives Ina May Gaskin and Sheila Kitzinger, for bringing back hands-on birthing! Thank you for the wonderful books you have given my students and me.

Mary Sharpe and Mary McMillan, for their groundbreaking work that made it easy to be birthing in good hands. I always think of Mary Sharpe, presently the director of the Midwifery Education Program at Ryerson University, as the Mother of Canadian Midwifery, and Mary McMillan, known as the Mother of Physical Therapy, who started work in England in the early 1900s and finished teaching at Harvard in the United States. Two Marys, two mothers of a special kind.

Jennifer Worth, for bringing *Call the Midwife* into the lives of men and women in 2018.

Grace Chan, for all the support over the years of working together, from our first meeting at the 3HO School of Massage in 1976 and then starting the Sutherland-Chan School and Teaching Clinic. Thanks, Grace, for being there at Crystal's birth and seeing me through a scary time. You were the best midwife I could have had!

Sarah Yarwood, English doula extraordinaire, photographer, videographer, production assistant, teaching assistant, labor and delivery partner, travel organizer, and writing babysitter. Couldn't have done Guatemala or this book without you!

Colleen Driscoll, maternity nurse and Dream Team partner in labor and delivery. Thank you for all your referrals over the years—Nadine especially! Thank you for those writing times together in your kitchen.

Ilene Bell, midwife dream come true, for coming to Nelson and integrating my life between Toronto and the West. Thank you for Apple Tree Maternity, my favorite teaching place in my hometown.

Catherine Ruskin: Toronto and Nelson meet in your wonderful midwifery. Thank you for Sharon and Sussi in Toronto and all our births in Nelson—you have enriched my experience immeasurably.

Dr. Ray Lake, Dr. Caroline Bennett, and Dr. Jean Memoreo: thank you for all your pregnant patients in Toronto and baby deliveries over the years. I loved delivering with all of you and especially Ray's boys. I learned so much from those Christmas holiday deliveries all those years ago. Women's College Hospital is the source of some of my favorite birthing memories. Thanks for bringing me up the right way, especially with those C-section miracles!

Dr. Svet Gueorjev and Dr. Jim Noiles, for your humor and expertise in the C-section department. Thank you for including me, hands on, with your patients.

Dr. Ken Muth, for your years of experience that make my patients feel safe in your hands. Listening to you and Dr. Gueorjev debate your expertise in stitches was an education to my patient and me during the aftermath of her C-section!

Dr. Lisa Sawyer, Dr. Janet Boyd, and Annabelle Sproule, for the latest hands-on tips for stretching the unstretchable! We are so lucky to have you all on the birthing team in Nelson.

Tracy Hill, for your co-teaching and training with me. Your patience and steady hands are such a gift to those you teach and treat. Good luck in your new nursing career!

Joni Bund, for your experience with goose grease massages and all your wild baby stories in between. Thank you for all the shoulder massages along the manuscript way—your touch saved my life many times!

Sarilyn Zimmerman, whose influence stays with me, in my stories and in my future. You were at that first birth with Judy more than forty years ago, and thank you today for keeping midwifery moving in Canada. I always boast about knowing you!!

Judy Pustil (postmortem), who is written into the roots of my school, my hometown, and my first birth. Thank you for all the love and support you gave Grace and me in attending our school and graduating in our first class.

Will Anielewicz, for your enthusiasm in producing my first maternity massage shoots in 1982 with Crystal, first pregnancy massage shoots in 1984 with Debra, and my first Down's syndrome baby massage production in 1985.

Debra and Fernando Forcello, for starring in my first traditional pregnancy massage video. Your film continues to show how to massage, thirty years later!

Sussi, Sofia, and Asha: thanks for all the shooting, everywhere and anywhere in Toronto that allowed me to spread my message of hands-on healing at our pet shoots and the high school massage for seniors shoots. You helped me bridge that gap between youth and seniors through the power of touch. Special thanks to your mother, Lona, our grandmother on the shoots, for her wonderful enthusiasm and support.

Krystal and her mom, Madeleine Greely, for being my first Down's syndrome film shoot, providing education to pass along for years to come—thanks again.

Claire Janz and baby friend Uri: thank you for the great filming and the wonderful continuation of the tactile talent you bring to all the public massage giveaways! Thank you also for introducing yourself to Uri's parents with "I'm Claire and I have Down's syndrome like your son, Uri." I wish I had a camera running for your narrative that day! You are a treasure.

Camara, for your story of loss and the enormous tribute you pay to your departed baby girl. You hold her in your heart so that we can all love her forever. If you hadn't asked Jill Beulieu for massages for Anaya as she crossed the rainbow bridge, we would have never met.

Nadine Boyd and Leesa Dean—my two wonderful (now both pregnant) literary twins.

Don Grayston and Ginger Shaw, for all your love, trust, and support when we met at Sorrento in 1970 and when I went to film school. Your social activism course shaped the curriculum at Sutherland Chan because you taught me the value of experiential learning, hands on.

Dr. Kevin McKechnie, for the inspiration of coaching each contraction. You are like an echo as you coach your laboring mothers, and a welcome addition to the heavenly birthing team at Kootenay Lake Hospital.

The Birthing Centre and Dr. Glen Hamill at Peace River Hospital in Fort St. John: thank you for the wonderful coaching and teaching opportunities in your unit, especially head nurse Kathleen Julian for organizing my classes. The highest birth rate in the country is well earned by you folks!

Holly, Rob, and Hazel, for the best YouTube results! Half a million viewers have watched you learn maternity massage. Thank you for being so easy to film.

Alison, Neco, baby Abby, and the entire clan of Wallach baby supporters: our military maternity massage and Christmas outdoor pregnancy shoot was one of my very funny favorites! Neco has the touch!

Wilma Boyd, our *Glamour* grandmother: thank you for your great delivery and hands-on skills showing how to massage your daughter, Nadine. You blew out the lights with your touch and your on-camera personality and demeanor!

Sebastian, massaging his baby sister Frances, and Chevy's two boys, massaging their baby sister. Chevy and Nadine: you brought up your boys to love massage. Their sisters have been under the influence of a touch that will change the world.

Max, Lindsay, Misty, and family: thank you for bringing touch into Max's recovery model. Your family is redesigning the world of special needs with your loving touch and therapeutic massage. Go Max go!!

Dénali, Selena, and Julie: *Two Moms and a Baby Girl: A Love Story* has been a wonderful experience for me in my professional and personal life. Your maternity massage, baby massage, and postpartum experience fueled the film. And then Lindsay and Dénali massaging Max helped me take the power of touch to the streets.

Dave, for your wonderful photos and your ongoing love for Dénali.

Lauri, my editor with Brush Education, for your undying patience and insistence on a finish. It was a pleasure to work with such a dynamic company and especially with you and your coaching skills to get me over the finish line.

My wonderful shooting team of Chris and Wyatt: thank you for your instant response to urgent calls for help! Two young men learning all the maternity insider information make for a changed world. Your ability to make our women and kids comfortable is so professional and appreciated! Many thanks to Valhalla Visuals!

Dan Caverly and Brian: your ladders and angles have made my films memorable, especially our musical massage with Loreena McKennitt, and the footage of Mary Colletti's incredible massage team in *Massaging Mary: Hands-on with ALS*. You made that film priceless with your shots of Ethan's concentration and gift of touch clearly in the viewers' experience.

Elizabeth Cunningham, Doug Jameson, and Emily: thank you. Elizabeth, thank you for asking me to tutor you all those years ago when we were twenty-five, helping you study in my very first teaching gig with the 3HO School of Massage in Toronto.

Annie and Dave, for your extended family: thank you for including me in your support team, with your sister Irene's births and Dénali's arrival. You are the best special parents for the boys and Dénali! They are touched forever by your love! Thank you for your photography talents over the years of documenting my life and my work.

Irene, for the deliveries of the boys, Mattie, Jacob, and Mitchell. Birthing your family with Annie was a dream come true. Raising your athletes with the practicalities of massage helps change the world.

Jill, for all the literary support, listening and keeping the fire stoked as I wrote the final chapters through the snowy winter in Ymir. Our Tuesdays of writing and massaging my hands kept me going through the tough last days. Your social worker skills have always helped my problems dissolve . . . remember to pray! Thank you for your practical skills with all the film shoots and organizing footage and cataloguing the work. But your touch saved my shoulders and hands many times, in this last year especially! Thank you, thank you, thank you.

Brandon, for the devotion and hands-on help when your sister was dying. The musical talent you are well known for will be surpassed with your hands-on skills with massage. Thank you for being on Bridget's team as she died, and thank you for the wonderful medical illustrations throughout the baby massage section of this book.

Francis Key, wherever you are: thank you for the treatment manual you did for me and for the students of Sutherland Chan. There had never been a teaching manual with such wonderful illustrations before. You were a gem to work with over those years of organizing massage strokes!

Fiona Rafferty and Maggie Mann, for being graduates of the Sutherland-Chan School and Teaching Clinic, for working with Grace and me in our first downtown clinic on Bay Street, and for changing the world of massage therapy training with your textbooks, now used all over the world.

Debra Curtis and Trish Dryden, for continuing excellence in massage therapy training and clinical practicums, and especially for your book *Breast Massage*. Trish, thank you for including me in your maternity experience, graduating in our first innovative evening medical professionals program, and for taking the bar higher with all your work at the levels of provincial and college certification in massage therapy. Debra, thank you for your partnership with Grace to elevate the reputation of Sutherland-Chan over the past twenty years, and for continuing to change the world of massage therapy training with your textbooks and Curtis Publishing.

My US editorial team of supporters, hands on with feedback and track changes and time spent writing beside me on your own projects.

Holly, for the Write a Novel in November start-off. Thank goodness for that conversation in the intersection outside the library. Your license plate said Texas and I just had to stop in mid-flight to compliment you for my extraordinary experience teaching with Grace in Texas years ago. When I saw that you were pregnant, we became instant friends; when I found out you were a writer, gainfully employed, I was in your kitchen every day, writing across the table from you!

Peter Schram, for being my longest-running shooter from pet massage to the *Magic of Massage* television series. You are a great shooter.

Our team leader, Jasmine Georget, for Write a Novel in November, during which I got my first 35,000 words on paper!

My writing team in Toronto; Lisa Ross in Kaslo; Natalka Podstawskyl, Elizabeth Cunningham, Colleen Driscoll, Linda Moore, Tom Wayman, Verna Relkoff, Andromeda Drake, Anne Degrace, and Nikki Barkley in Nelson.

My pregnant couples in Nelson and Toronto. Forty years ago with Judy and John Knibb and Rebecca MacKenzie and Dan; forty days ago with Brady and Tasha and their wonderful partners.

Laura Repo Davis for taking over my niche in Toronto so I could come home to BC. Thank you for all your mother and baby work in Toronto with Go Slow Mama.

My summer maternity class during this book's gestation: Kim Knox, Eugenie Brusa, Amanda Phoenix, Nahimsa Elmahir, Melissa Cataford, Maya Barkley, Sydnee Paavola, Eleanor Tweddell, Sarah Yarwood, and Jacklyn Banman.

Le Linh in Vietnam, who got me started teaching globally through Skype. Thank you for your enthusiasm and all the pregnant teams who came to the clinic every week for Maternity Mondays teaching in Vietnam!

Nahima Elmahir, for your wonderful organizational skill and attention to detail. You made teaching in Haiti at the Olive Tree Birthing Center the best!

Melinda and Susan from Ellison's Market, for supporting Nahima's Canada tour with your vegetables, and my Haiti tour with your inspirational stories of the Olive Tree Birthing Centre.

Staff at the Haiti Arise Complex, for organizing my teaching and bringing all the pregnant people for my classes. Thank you to Nelson Rotary for their support of the project.

Erin and her mother, for giving me my first experience with an adoptive birth. It was a sacred passage of touch. Thank you for helping my summer maternity students learn to extend their hearts and hands as well.

George Coton, for the hours of helping my final edits and great literary coaching, especially at three in the morning.

Ron Vankoughnett, for his coaching to help me find my voice and speak up.

Hopi Glockner, for the help over the years from when you were a child until now, as a doula in your own right. You have the touch!

Harrison, Tristan, and Ashton, for your enthusiasm in massaging your pregnant mother and your help with the flash-mob massages on Boxing Day at the hospital. Thanks also to your parents, Alison and Brian, for raising you with touch as a positive force in your home life.

The many families and students who taught me how to teach: thank you for your feedback and enthusiasm for birthing in good hands.

My parents, Margaret and Bill Sutherland, for teaching me family values and allowing me to employ my birthing skills in their lives and in their passing. You gave me a gift in the high value of hand holding, and the comfort of touch.

My daughter, Crystal Anielewicz, for your wonderful photography talent on the beautiful book cover and your pregnancy photo shoots. Thank you also for bringing massage into your professional world with high school kids massaging seniors. You have bridged the gap that will allow both your kids and the seniors of your community to feel the love through touch and massage. Thank you for all your work in the policies you are creating in the LGBTQ two-spirited community; you are bridging a gap that will bring healing where it is most needed. You are a wonderful daughter and a great team player. Thank you.

INDEX

ABOUT THE AUTHOR

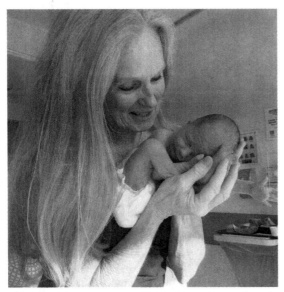

Christine welcomes a twin, still curled from the womb, to the world, 2016.

Christine Sutherland is a filmmaker, author, and registered massage therapist. Her latest books, *Dying in Good Hands* and *Birthing in Good Hands*, are massage inspirations to teach both the medical professional and layperson to alleviate pain and increase comfort during two of life's major transitions. She makes Nelson, British Columbia, her home base as she travels the world spreading her message of hands-on healing.

Christine started the Sutherland-Chan School of Massage Therapy with her former student from the 3HO School of Massage, Grace Chan, in 1978.

In her career since that time, she has toured with musicians all over Europe and North America, worked with Olympic and wheelchair athletes, and helped in many types of deliveries, including horses, cows, and humans.

Teaching massage to others is her passion, and the global classroom is her venue, from studying in Germany at the Kneipp School to teaching midwives in a 120-family collective of Guatemalan freedom fighters. She's staged "flash-mob" massage events at local hospitals and other events to teach people how to share a healing touch. Her favorite massage activity is "Bridging the Gap" in which she teaches youth to massage seniors in Canada and, using computer technology, as far afield as Africa, Haiti, and Guatemala. Christine's YouTube channel teaches 24/7 with more than a half million views of her films for all stages of maternity and baby massage, wheelchair massage, palliative massage, and pet massage.

From Christine's first baby delivery in the backcountry of northern Ontario in 1977 to the pool birth in Nelson last week, the magic of massage has played along those forty years of labor and love. Find Christine at www.christinesutherland.com.

Facebook: https://www.facebook.com/ChristineLSutherland/

YouTube: https://www.youtube.com/user/SutherlandMassage